For The Duration

To Daphne Malins
from a friend of
the author.
  Elsa Grandi
June 29. 1997

For The Duration

Eve Porter Jacobsen

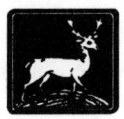

Pentland Press, Inc.
United States of America

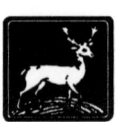

PUBLISHED BY PENTLAND PRESS, INC.
5124 Bur Oak Circle, Raleigh, North Carolina 27612
United States of America
919-782-0281

ISBN 1-57197-006-1
Library of Congress Catalog Card Number 95-69540

Copyright © 1995 Eve Porter Jacobsen
All rights reserved, which includes the right to reproduce this book or portions thereof in any form whatsoever except as provided by the U.S. Copyright Law.

Printed in the United States of America

To Dorothy Floyd Rutter
who has been my best friend since
we were small children and always will be.

Chapter One

From all accounts I must have been a very boring little girl, for when approached by strangers, I would cling, howling, to Mother's skirts. The first night I ever spent away from home was a sad mistake. I was four years old and had looked forward so much to spending a night at Aunt Edith's big house and sharing a room with Cousin Helen, but an exasperated Uncle Ted, who looked as though he might be suffering from acute insomnia, thankfully took me home as soon as it was light.

Mother scolded me. "Eve," she said, "I'm ashamed of you! You're a big girl now." But I was safe at home and that was all that mattered to me.

Actually Cousin Helen was to blame. She was then nine years old and already had the makings of a future know-it-all and was terribly anxious to impress her small cousin with all the remarkable knowledge she was gaining at school. One of the things she told me was that the whole world was going round and round all the time and what had haunted me all night was the thought that the piece of world with Mother in it might move around faster than the piece I was in and that I might never catch up with her.

It looked as though I would be a girl tied and devoted to home life always, and in all probability I would have been, had not a certain man in Germany named Adolf Hitler had ideas about world leadership. Now, looking back across the years, I can hardly believe that I have been to so many places and met so many people. I have had sweet nothings whispered into my responsive ear on moonlit decks in the Atlantic, Pacific, and Indian Oceans. I have thrown coins to gully-gully boys in Algiers, been fleeced by souvenir vendors in Egypt, ridden a smelly camel in Aden, been almost drowned in the swimming pool at the once-famous Poona Club, and viewed night life from all angles in Calcutta. I have been pursued by a romantic Spaniard in the Dutch West Indies, flung out of a jeep in Jamaica, and been almost burned alive in New Zealand. I have been spellbound by the beauty of Sydney Harbor, the wildness of the New Guinea jungle, and the quiet grandeur of the Canadian Rockies.

Travel did not play a major part during my early life, largely because of my disconcerting habit of always being disgustingly sick in cars, trains, and buses, but I am completely cured of that. In fact the cure is so complete that I have since dined heartily in an almost deserted dining saloon in a choppy sea in the Bay of Biscay.

I was fourteen the first time I was taken to London and I was not impressed. Crossing the streets was a nightmare and the tube trains made my head ache. Londoners, I thought, were much too gushing after the cautious reserve of my Yorkshire contemporaries. So, it was with a feeling of relief that after two weeks of frantic rush and bustle, I left London, hoping that I would never have to go again, but I did. The Ministry of Labor took care of that during the war which was to follow so soon, and that is where my story begins.

I know that if I live to be a hundred I shall never forget that sunny Sunday morning, September 3, 1939, for it was on that morning for the first time in my life, I experienced terror—real terror. It was really terror of the unknown for in the years that followed I was to have much more terrifying experiences, but they came upon me gradually and I became adjusted to them.

I spent the last two weeks of the school holidays that summer at the home of my friend, Dorothy Floyd, in Northumberland. The Floyds had previously lived near us in Scarborough and Dorothy and I had been friends all our lives. Our mothers were great friends too.

Usually the Floyd household was a very lively one, but Noel, the elder son, was in the Royal Naval Volunteer Reserve and was called up for service. He, of course, was wildly excited about going—what eighteen-year-old wasn't in those days?

But I knew how Mrs. Floyd cried and cried after he had marched off so proudly in his uniform to God alone knew what. Maurice, the younger son, who was then nearly seventeen, was longing for the day when he could join up too. Dorothy and I were somewhat bewildered by all that was going on.

The sun shone brilliantly through the wide-open windows as we—Mrs. Floyd, Dorothy, Maurice, and I—gathered round the radio to hear Mr. Chamberlain's announcement at eleven o'clock. Mr. Floyd was not at home, having left shortly before to call on Mr. Howlett, a business acquaintance.

It had been expected, but to actually hear the prime minister say, "and that consequently this country is at war with Germany," was a dreadful shock. With tears rolling down her cheeks, Mrs. Floyd switched off the radio.

Maurice was the first to break the silence that followed. "Gosh!" he said, "I hope it goes on long enough for me to get into it."

His mother said, "Maurice, you're not to talk like that! It will all be over before Christmas. I know it will."

Hardly were the words out of her mouth when the air raid warning sounded. We gazed helplessly at each other then Mrs. Floyd, taking command of the situation, said, "We'd better go to your father. Hurry!"

Looking back at that mad panic now almost makes me want to laugh. In the years that were to follow, Britain certainly proved to the whole world that she could "take it" but on the occasion of that first warning—which turned out to be a false alarm—a large majority of us made absolute fools of ourselves. Mrs. Floyd made a wild dash for insurance policies, Dorothy got out her gas mask and was about to put it on when Maurice stopped her.

"You don't need to put it on, you silly idiot," he said with brotherly candor. "That wasn't a gas warning." Then, although the weather was warm, he got coats for all of us and I combed my hair—why, I will never know. Leaving the front door unlocked—"those beastly Germans will break it in anyway"—we tore up the street. Various neighbors were standing in their front gardens gazing up at the sky. One man asked Dorothy where we were going.

"We are going to my father, so that we can all die together," she said idiotically.

We were half way along Mayville Avenue when Mrs. Floyd suddenly realized that she was wearing hair curlers and there was another moment of panic. Air raid or no air raid, she could not possibly go to the Howletts in hair curlers, so out they came and were scattered in the roadway as we dashed madly along. I still blush when I think of it all.

We ran up the drive to the Howletts' front door and found the porch piled high with sandbags. The side door was also piled with sandbags and finally we made an entry via the kitchen where, for the first time that morning, we laughed. Peggy and Milly, the cook and housemaid, with cushions on their heads, were sitting at the table shelling peas.

"It's for the blast," they explained.

We went through the hall to the drawing room where Mrs. Howlett sat stiffly in regal splendor, wearing a blue velvet cushion on her head and rolling bandages for the Red Cross. "It's for the blast," she said.

Mr. Howlett and Mr. Floyd were strutting around in tin hats looking very important.

It was not long before the "all clear" sounded and Mr. Floyd took us all home.

"Well, we have come through our first air raid without a scratch," Dorothy said complacently. What a blessing we did not know then what was ahead of us or how long the war would last—before it was over, Dorothy and I would both become nurses and that Maurice would lie in a soldier's grave near Benghazi.

The next day I went home. Mrs. Floyd saw me safely onto the train and Mother met me at the station. I was so pleased to see her that I almost hugged the breath out of her. I felt as though she alone could protect me from any of the horrors that Hitler might think of. There was nothing in our dear little seaside town for Hitler to want anyway. But on the way home I realized that the authorities thought differently—even here the buildings were sandbagged, air raid warning notices were everywhere and all along the sea front, which was usually crowded with holiday-makers at this time of the year, were barbed wire entanglements, and huge concrete blocks had been erected in the roadway. I felt sick inside as I surveyed it all—it seemed somehow to be the end of my childhood, yet I did not feel grown-up. However, I was home and there I felt safe.

Things were just as usual except that all the windows now had anti-blast strapping on them and an Anderson shelter had been constructed in the garden. My brothers, who were older than I—Arthur twenty-two and Reg twenty-seven, and my father were enthusiastically fitting it out with all manner of comforts and escape devices. Fortunately we did not need to use the shelter at all that winter. By Christmas the "phony war" as it was called, had been on for three months and although food was rationed there were no real shortages as yet.

We had our usual lively Christmas with the house being full at all times with relatives and friends. My brothers and most of their friends were expecting to be called up in the New Year as they had volunteered one after the other for various branches of the armed forces.

In the spring of 1940, things really began to happen. The low countries were invaded one after the other. Many, many bombs fell on Britain. Our shipping losses—thanks to Hitler's magnetic mine—were fantastic; there was the miracle of Dunkirk and then France capitulated.

I was on my way home from school when I heard about France. Two workmen were discussing it in the street and I couldn't help overhearing them. I quickened my footsteps.

"Mummy, is France really out of the war?" I asked as soon as I burst through the front door.

"Yes," she said quietly, then seeing how white I was, she put her arms about me. "Don't worry, darling," she comforted me. "At least we know now where we stand and thank God this is an island and we have the finest navy in the world." Dear, dear Mummy—she always made me feel so secure.

It was not Hitler's plan, at first, to bomb London. It seemed he wanted to march in triumph through an undamaged capital. "Surround London, but do not attack," he ordered the Luftwaffe. "Starve her people." It was his intention to destroy our cities one by one and Coventry was the first but by no means the last. Many big cities were bombarded again and again and continuous attacks were made on the airfields of Sussex and Kent, but it was not until August that Hitler turned his attention to London and her vast cities. There were only occasional raids at first and we retaliated by bombing Berlin. This was not easy because of the great distance our planes had to travel to reach the target, but for the Germans to travel from their bases in occupied France it was no problem at all.

After the bombing of Berlin it became obvious that Hitler wanted revenge and the bombing of London was intensified—his aim now was to destroy London completely. His target had switched from airfields and armament factories, to the people, homes, hospitals, and schools in London. It was, however, Hitler's greatest error, for the people of London were undaunted and while London bled, armament output in the provinces increased.

Hitler had also underestimated the Royal Air Force. There were three thousand Nazi planes against nine hundred British fighter planes, but for every British plane lost the Germans lost three and perhaps more, as British estimates of enemy losses were often understated.

German losses from daylight raids became so costly that the bombers came in the dark. However, our night-fighters who were soon equipped with air interception equipment, or radar as we now call it, reigned supreme. Also, Winston Churchill was now Prime Minister.

By this time things had changed considerably at home. Reg, my elder brother, was in the army and Arthur, the younger one, was in the Royal Air Force (R.A.F.). The house seemed to be so strange and quiet without them and I began to feel very lonely.

Someone else who also seemed to be feeling lonely now that all his friends were drifting into the services was Donald

Bell. For as long as I could remember, Donald had been a friend of Reg's. He was now almost thirty and, as far as we knew, his age group would not be called up for several months.

"I really feel that I should volunteer the same as most of the other boys have done," he said to Mother one evening. "But I want to hang on as long as I can for Mother's sake." Donald's brothers and sisters were all married and his father had died only a few months before the war broke out.

"I don't blame you," Mother said. "We know that you will have to go eventually and it will be very hard for your mother, so let her get used to being without your father first."

In our loneliness, Donald and I drifted together that summer. He often helped me with my homework—he was a wizard at mathematics which I loved—and we played tennis frequently. We also went for long walks in the country. There were so many lovely spots all around us, and we took long walks along the cliffs. He could rarely use his car as gas was so strictly rationed.

Donald teased me a great deal just as my brothers had always done, but it was a different kind of teasing and I did not resent it the way I resented my brothers' teasing, and in his company I began to gain self-confidence which I knew I needed. He also encouraged me to talk about myself, about school, my ambitions, and everything that interested me and of course we discussed the war all the time. I knew he was longing to go into the Royal Navy and, as conscription for women was now in operation and as it looked as though the war might last for a long time, we speculated on what I should join eventually.

Reg came home on leave that Christmas in 1940 and was married to his sweetheart, Nell. It was a quiet wedding, as most weddings were in those days, but it was a very pretty one. Since it was winter, Nell wanted an all velvet wedding with her in white velvet and the bridesmaids, Carol Walters and me, in red velvet.

"They want me to wear red velvet," I fumed to Donald when I saw him. "Carol will look wonderful and I'll look awful."

"How come?" he asked.

"I can't wear red," I said. "Instead of giving me color it just makes me look paler than ever. Can you imagine me beside Carol—pale, skinny and ugly?"

"Come, come now. I won't have that," Donald broke in. Donald laughed. He was always laughing, that's why he had such deep lines around his eyes. "Who says you are all these things?" he asked.

I pouted. "You know Arthur always calls me 'skinny Lizzie,'" I said.

"I know that, but he's only teasing. Anyway he's your brother. I know what brothers are. I should—I've been one all my life. Now let's look at this seriously. What did you say you are—pale, skinny and ugly? Shame on you." He looked quizzically at me. "Let's say instead, fair, petite and—when you learn how to use those big blue eyes—very attractive, especially when you blush as you are doing now."

"Don't be silly," I said.

"Now my child, that is one thing you will have to learn—how to accept a compliment," Donald said seriously. "Don't shuffle and say, 'don't be silly.' It seems to me I had better take you in hand and help you to become a poised sophisticated woman of the world." I wasn't sure whether he was teasing me or not.

"What's this about Carol looking wonderful?" he asked.

"Well you know she has such lovely dark curls and smooth creamy skin. Red is her color all right," I said.

"She also has thin lips and thick ankles," Donald replied. "But you my pet are too young and naive to notice it yet. Now as soon as you get a snippet of that red velvet we'll go out and buy a lipstick to match."

"Mummy won't let me use lipstick," I said.

Donald patted my shoulder. "I'll have a word with her about that," he promised.

Apparently Donald knew what he was talking about because I loved my red velvet dress and so many people told me I looked nice in it.

One of the guests at the wedding was John Glennie. I had not seen him for some time as he was at Cambridge, but I had known him all my life and for the past year or so I had

had quite a crush on him. I think Donald guessed it and he made sure that John and I got together at the reception. John was most attentive, and after complimenting me on my appearance asked me if I would like to go dancing at the Grand Hotel that night.

I was afraid that Mother would say no, even though she liked John, but Donald came to the rescue again. He suggested a foursome and invited Cousin Helen to partner him. This was a very noble effort on his part. I knew he did not really like her. She had grown into a great beauty, but she was an aggressive, self-opinionated bore.

It was so exciting being taken out to my first dance at the "Grand" with a tall good-looking "older man"—John was almost twenty-one—and I loved every minute of it.

He was a good dancer and he complimented me on my dancing. How thankful I was that when Arthur had been taking ballroom dancing lessons he had needed someone to practice with at home.

After the dance Donald and Helen went home in Donald's car, but John and I decided to walk home. It was a glorious night with a brilliant moon—how we loved moonlight on those grim nights of complete blackout—and unusually mild for December.

We walked across the beach and sat for a while on the steps of an old bathing hut. John said quietly, "I've been accepted for the R.A.F. I expect I'll be getting my papers pretty soon."

"You are all going away one by one," I said. There always seemed to be so little to say on these occasions.

There was a pause and then he said, "Eve, will you write to me when I go away?"

I said I would like to very much. "You're such a sweet kid," he said and he kissed me for the first time as we sat there on the steps of the old bathing hut.

After he went into the R.A.F., John's letters were a great comfort to me for in February we learned the shattering news that Mother had only a few months to live. I was a coward and refused to accept it. Mother had always been my idol. I wanted to be like her in every way. Life without her was unthinkable, and I who had been spoiled and pampered all my life, hated to face facts. I poured out my heart to John in those letters—he was the only one I felt I could discuss it with and he was so wonderful about everything.

He came home on leave twice that year and we began to make plans for the future—or as much of the future as one dared to think about in those days. He had just gone back from leave in September when Mother died, but he helped me through that dreadful period when we knew the end was very near.

Dad and I carried on as well as we could after Mother died. Lucy, our hardworking and always willing "daily help" then left us to join the Auxiliary Territorial Service.

There were tears in her eyes when she told us she was leaving us. "I feel terrible about leaving you at a time like this," she said. "But if I wait till they call me up, they'll make an army cook of me I know and I want to go on the ack-ack guns and have a crack at them rotten Germans."

In December John wrote to say that he hoped to get Christmas leave. "I should have my wings by then," he wrote, but he was killed on December 21.

It seemed there were no words to comfort me. His death had achieved nothing; he had not even killed one enemy. He had crashed on his final training flight—so, he got his wings for Christmas.

That Christmas was the unhappiest of my life. For each other's sake, Dad and I made an effort to celebrate Christmas. Friends invited us to spend Christmas Day with them but for the remainder of the week I just moped. Then, on New Year's Eve, Donald insisted on taking me out and we went to the Gala Dance at the Royal Hotel—I was so grateful that he did not suggest the Grand Hotel.

He tried hard to make the evening a happy one and I tried too. On the stroke of midnight, I obediently joined hands as everyone sang "Auld Lang Syne." I tried to sing too but I felt that my heart was breaking and Donald seemed to understand.

Quietly and unobtrusively, he led me out to a balcony and led me to a seat there. I put my head in my hands and cried quietly while Donald leaned on the parapet and smoked a cigarette.

Some time later, he came over and sat beside me. "Feeling better now?" he asked. I nodded and he gave me his handkerchief. "Have a good blow," he said.

Obediently I did as I was told, then, cupping my chin in his hands, he kissed me on the lips. "Happy New Year," he said softly.

"Happy New Year, Donald," I said.

"And now come and look at this lovely view," he said. "I don't think we ever really appreciated it when we had all that artificial lighting in peace time." We leaned on the parapet and watched the waves breaking on the dark shore. It was very beautiful.

"The old year hasn't been a very happy one for you, has it, Eve?" he said quietly. "I'll bet you feel that you have really grown up now, don't you?"

I nodded. I couldn't trust myself to speak.

"That's one of the awful things about war," he went on, "especially for anyone as young as you. Years from now you will probably wonder just what did happen to your youth. Seventeen should be such a happy, carefree year for a girl but for you, it has taken away your mother and your first sweetheart. You know of course, that you can never get another mother, but John won't be your last sweetheart. Now, don't interrupt," he said as I made a motion to do so. "I'm sure you think now that no one could possibly take John's place but time will tell. In future years, many men will adore you, I feel absolutely sure about that. I don't know just what it is about you, Eve, but there's an underlying quality about you that brings out the best in men, so don't be bitter, please. You have so much ahead of you—I feel it in my bones, really. Tell me now that you will try hard to overcome this awful tragedy and, if it's at all possible, to benefit from the experience. Promise?"

"Yes, Donald, I promise," I whispered.

I really meant it, and, as Donald stood there and held my hand during those first few moments of 1942, I knew that I had left youth behind me, that I was ready to take my place as a grown-up in this war-shattered country of mine.

Chapter Two

In those days, it seemed to me that people became immune to grief and shock, and I was no exception. In February of 1942 my father went to Hull on a business trip and had a fatal heart attack, but I hardly shed a tear. The only home I had ever known was gone and I went to stay with Aunt Edith and Uncle Ted. It was a lonely existence for me there; even Helen was gone. She had become a junior officer in the Auxiliary Territorial Service. A huge photograph of her in her army uniform held a place of honor in the living room and her boastful letters were always read aloud by Aunt Edith.

Helen came home on her first ten-day leave soon after I went to live there. I must admit that she looked really stunning in her uniform. Most women looked drab in khaki, but not Helen. With her blond hair and flawless, creamy skin, her tall well-proportioned figure and her clear blue eyes, she looked like a Viking goddess. Without a blush, she told me often and at great length what an asset she was to the British army. I was so relieved when she finally went off to rejoin her unit because I was getting worried about the state the war office must be in during her absence.

A turning point came in my life a few months after Dad died. The Floyds offered me a home with them for as long as I wanted to stay. Naturally, I accepted as the Floyds were the only people with whom I really wanted to be. Aunt Edith was rather tearful when I told her, but I think that underneath she was greatly relieved. Only conscience had prompted her to take me in the first place, certainly not affection.

I felt much happier after I went to live with the Floyds. Dorothy and I had been friends all our lives and we had so much in common—even our frequent squabbles were fun. We joined the British Red Cross Society, attended lectures and studied together. We made our first uniforms ourselves and after getting our first aid and home nursing certificates, we proudly stitched red crosses on our aprons. At first we did voluntary part-time work in a local emergency hospital, but as we became more and more absorbed in nursing we decided to take it up full-time, for the duration, and went on the payroll.

We were still having occasional air raids, but not on the scale we had known them in 1940 and 1941. They were mostly hit and run raids now. We had learned to take them in stride by this time just as we had learned to live with blackouts and food shortages. Maybe nursing was my salvation. I worked hard and became tired so that I was able to sleep even through air raids, and eventually I was able to put my heartache into the background.

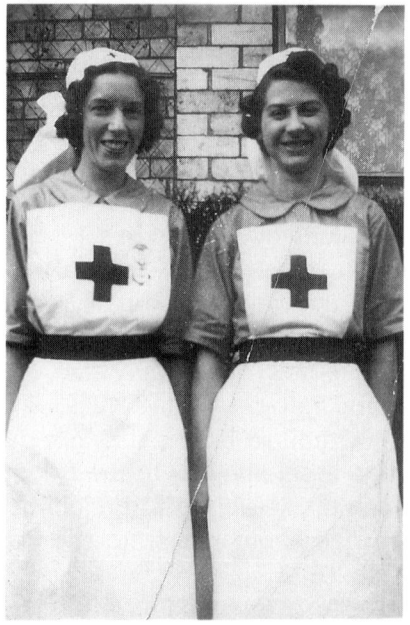
Eve and Dorothy

The church we attended opened a canteen for troops and Dorothy and I often gave assistance there when we were off duty from the hospital. We brought many lonely servicemen home where, somehow, Mrs. Floyd always managed to stretch the rations and feed them. It was also at church that I met David. He was twelve years my senior and very eligible, so I was naturally very flattered when he began to take an interest in me. He was in a reserved occupation at the shipyard and although he wanted to join the Royal Navy, he was not allowed to do so.

Maurice, Dorothy's brother, joined the army that year and took to it as a duck takes to water. When he came home on leave we could hardly take our eyes off him—he was so tall and broad and so very tough. Was this our gentle aesthetic Maurice?

It was in September that I decided to become a mobile Voluntary Aid Detachment (V.A.D.). I was still in the Red Cross but as a V. A. D. nurse I came under military law and could be sent anywhere. Previously I had only worn the indoor Red Cross uniform but now I had to be measured for the outdoor uniform and I was very pleased with the result. The navy blue jacket and skirt fitted me perfectly and I proudly stitched my "mobile" badge to the left sleeve.

I was posted to a hospital in North London. Prior to the war it had been a children's orthopedic hospital but the children had long since been transferred to a place of comparative safety in the country and the hospital had been serving as an emergency hospital since then.

I was not too happy about being posted to London as I had not liked it when I went there as a child, but this of course was a vastly different London. It was a city devastated by war, fighting desperately. I was proud to be in London at such a time and I came to love it with a fierce and patriotic devotion. It never failed to awe and inspire me and I became familiar with its history and romance, her narrow old-world streets and wide shopping thoroughfares, its heartbreaking battle scars and its wonderful transport system which, even in wartime, was second to none.

I also became familiar with those gallant men and women who made up London's Air Raid Precautions Service, the heroic policemen and firemen, the ambulance drivers, who had to drive their vehicles through pitch darkness where bombs were falling and where there were often great craters in the roads, and the way everyone carried on against such alarming odds with amazing cheerfulness.

To London I gave what are fondly believed by many to be the "best years of one's life" and I paid for it in blood and toil, tears and sweat, just as our wonderful prime minister had promised. I worked harder than I had believed anyone could work, but deep down, I loved it.

I always spent my leaves with the Floyds where I always found love, kindness, warmth and a veritable haven of rest. Noel, their elder son, was somewhere around the coast of India and in the late summer of that year Maurice was drafted to Egypt. Dorothy was still working in the local hospital and became engaged to Al Rutter, a young soldier whom she had met at church.

I think Mrs. Floyd had fond hopes of pairing me off with David, once she had recovered from the shock of learning about the twelve-year difference in our ages. David looked so ridiculously young that it was hard for anyone to believe that he was thirty. I must admit that I became very fond of him. He was such a staunch, reliable person and no matter what hour of the day or night I arrived, he always managed to be at the station to await my arrival, often at great inconvenience to himself, especially when trains were delayed as they so often were during the war. Whatever I wanted I could have and, I regret to say, I came to take him far too much for granted.

I managed to get Christmas leave that year and although it was almost two o'clock in the morning when I arrived, and snowing heavily, dear David was there waiting for me in spite of the fact that he had to be at work in five hours.

By this time food had really become a major problem but somehow we managed to have a reasonably festive spread. The absence of the two boys naturally cast something of a shadow, but we said, "Maybe next Christmas it will be over and we can all be together again." We did not know exactly where Noel was but we did know that Maurice was safe at a base camp in Egypt. It was on the last day of my leave that the blow fell.

I was awakened about half past eight that morning by a piercing scream. I jumped out of bed and flew along the landing. Mrs. Floyd ran up the stairs and flinging herself in my arms, she sobbed and sobbed and sobbed. Maurice had been killed.

"Oh, dear God, when is all this slaughter going to end," I asked myself.

Back at the hospital I found myself on night duty for three months and in a way I was glad. One does not need to laugh and talk quite so much on night duty, and for that I was thankful. I became despondent and on edge, found myself avoiding people. I began to hate nursing. I wanted to get out of it but knew there was no escape. I was in this for the duration. A fatigue and despair such as I had never known took possession of me. The emergency hospital was not a big one and the patients were a mixture of everything—navy, army, and air force personnel, civilians, chronically ill, and even on occasion, a few children.

One morning Cousin Helen paid me a surprise visit. She was as patronizing as ever and still the same old pain in the neck to me. It had been a hectic night on duty and the other three night nurses and I were almost speechless with fatigue as we pulled our capes tightly about us and set off from the hospital to the quarters in the cold morning air.

"Wonder what sort of poison they will dish up for us this morning," Micki Daniels said with a great yawn.

"Sausages as usual, I expect," Diana Bourne said in her singsong Welsh voice.

"The minute the war's over I shall eat myself sick," quiet Louise Adams said slowly.

"Not if you are in this place," I put in. "Barney wouldn't allow you."

"Oh, they'll pension Barney off before this lot's over!" Louise said, and we all laughed.

"Gosh it's cold," Diana said, trying to draw her small head down inside the collar of her cape.

We took off our capes in the vestibule of our quarters and filed into the dining room where the tightlipped Miss Barnes was presiding at the serving hatch. The blackout screens were still up on this cold dark morning and a weak yellow light illuminated the drab dining room.

"Where is your belt, Nurse Bourne?" Barney snapped in her husky, unpleasant voice. Barney never missed a thing. Muttering under her breath, Diana took the offending belt out of her pocket and put it on. "I don't know how many times you girls have been told never to come to meals improperly dressed," she rasped. There was much more of it. That was the worst of Barney. She would never let well enough alone.

Why the powers that be had put a nagging old harridan like her in charge of us we could never understand.

"Any news of leave yet?" Louise asked, anxious to change the subject. Louise was a privileged person. Being older than all of us, she was credited by Barney with having more sense.

"I expect Matron will put the list on the board this morning," Barney replied. "You aren't due for leave though, Nurse Porter," she added, fixing me with a glare.

"I'm quite aware of that," I said crisply.

"You've only been back from leave about six weeks," she said accusingly.

"Well, don't get excited. I'm not complaining," I said quietly, but I felt like shaking the stupid old woman.

"How about something to eat, Barney darling? We're simply starving," Micki said with a most angelic look on her beautiful face, but, I felt sure, with murder in her heart.

"I'm going as fast as I can. I've only got one pair of hands," the old battle-ax retorted.

Soon we found ourselves facing brown Windsor soup, a weird looking concoction of spam fried in batter, butter beans, and mashed potatoes. When I was on day duty it always nauseated me to see the night staff tucking away heavy dinners at eight o'clock in the morning, but when I was on night duty myself it seemed perfectly natural. As usual, when the meals were particularly revolting we fortified ourselves by discussing the things we would eat when the war ended.

With the meal finished, we trooped off to bed, yawning our heads off. Two boxy little rooms in the most remote corner of the building were allotted to the night staff. It was by no means quiet there but it was quieter than anywhere else and we usually managed to get a good day's sleep if we left the blackout screens up. Fortunately the screens had ventilation slats so we were permitted to leave them up.

Barney really liked us to go for a brisk walk before going to bed but she did not always get her own way on freezing cold mornings. This was one of those mornings. Micki and Diana were especially anxious to get to bed early this morning as they were getting up at two o'clock to go to a tea dance with two convalescent patients. None of us knew how they managed to get out without running into Barney but they never failed. The two of them were giggling together in the bathroom as my roommate Louise and I prepared for bed.

"I can't think where they get their energy," Louise said as she got out her clean uniform for the night. "This is the third time this week they have been out in the afternoon."

"It's amazing," I agreed. "I don't know how they can be bothered just to go out with a couple of patients. Not that I have anything against them, they are nice enough boys, but I don't know. I never fancied going out with patients somehow."

"Nor me. I prefer them healthy," Louise said with a laugh. "Lend me your head, will you, dear? I want to make up a cap." I sat down on the chair and she had just finished making up the cap when Barney waddled in.

"Nurse Porter—there's a visitor to see you downstairs," she said. "An A.T.S. (Auxiliary Territorial Service) officer."

"Cousin Helen," I groaned. "That's all I need."

"It's an awkward time to be visiting," Barney grumbled. "Don't let her stay too long. You ought to be getting some sleep."

Barney was still grumbling as we walked down the stairs. I felt like pushing her head first down the stairs but instead I put my arm around her plump shoulders.

"Listen, Barney dear," I said. "I didn't ask her to come and if you knew my Cousin Helen you would understand why, but if she hasn't gone in fifteen minutes be an angel and come and rescue me, will you?"

She promised that she would and I went into the sitting room to see Helen. Of course, the sight of Helen in her immaculate uniform which showed off her tall, splendid figure to perfection, reminded me of my smallness, my untidy hair, bedroom slippers and pale, tired face.

"Hullo, Helen. It's nice to see you," I lied.

"Darling, I'm sorry to come at such an ungodly hour," she gushed in her high, affected voice, "but I had to come to town on a *secret mission*." You could almost see the italics. "I knew you would never forgive me if I didn't find time to pop along and say hello."

"That's what you think," I said to myself. Out loud I said, "That's quite all right. I'm so glad I was not in bed. You timed it beautifully."

I noticed that she had another pip on her shoulder. "Why Helen, you are a junior commander now. How wonderful. Congratulations." I knew then why she had taken the trouble to come and see me and I hoped that I had hit on the correct rank. Apparently that was what A.T.S. three-pippers called themselves, otherwise she would have made no bones about correcting me.

She rattled on for what seemed hours about the war office, secret documents, King's Regulations, Northern Command and other jargon while I struggled to look intelligent and keep my eyes open. Even as a schoolgirl Helen had always been objectionable in my opinion, but as an A.T.S. officer she was even worse. Seeing her always put me in a bad temper and made me feel like the most hopeless failure. Listening to her prattling on about what a Godsend she was to the army made me wonder why they still went on enlisting hundreds more girls when they already had Cousin Helen. Downright extravagance, that's what it is, I thought. No wonder the war was costing so much money.

Presently she asked me how I was getting on in my "little job." She had always looked on my decision to become a Red Cross nurse with tolerant amusement. "I suppose it will be all right for you," she had said condescendingly, "but of course it would be no use for me. I must have action. I would hate taking orders from some of those ghastly ward sisters. Even at school I was always destined to be a leader." She was right about that. She had always been bossy.

For perhaps the first time in my life I was glad to see Barney waddle in officiously at the end of fifteen minutes or so. "Yes, I know what you are coming for," Helen said sweetly, "and I'm just going. Nurse looks so tired, doesn't she? Well, bye-bye, dear. You are doing a simply wonderful job."

When I went back upstairs Louise was already sound asleep, so I undressed as quietly as possible while my bath was running. Just as I knew it would, Helen's visit had brought on another fit of depression for me. Why had I taken on this rotten job, I wondered. There was nothing but hard work, long hours, horrors, sharp commands, long spells of night duty and hardly any pay.

"I'll desert—that's what I'll do," I said to myself as I slipped between the icy sheets and hugged my hot water bag. That must have been my last waking thought as it only seemed a few minutes later that I heard a loud banging on the door and Jean Lloyd yelling that it was time to get up.

She snapped on the light and bustled in carrying two cups of steaming tea. Louise, who awakened immediately, said, "Jean, you angel," and wrapping her hands about the hot cup sipped it gratefully. Rousing myself with difficulty I sat and took the remaining cup of delicious, thick, brown tea while Jean perched herself on the foot of my bed.

"The leave list went up today," she said excitedly. "I go on the twenty-second."

"Good," I said, hating at that moment any lucky creature who happened to be going home.

"You are not on the list," Jean said unabashed.

"Jean," I said, fixing her with one of my looks. "You are a dear sweet soul for bringing tea for us, but if you did it simply for the sake of barging in to break a piece of bad news and gloating over those less fortunate than yourself, I think you are an absolute stinker."

As usual Jean refused to be snubbed. "Darling," she cooed, "you know perfectly well that I always bring you a cup of tea on the days when I am off duty at five o'clock."

"Maybe so, but you always do it with greater gusto when you have any nauseating news or disgusting piece of gossip to impart," I replied.

"Well, I'm a woman, aren't I?" she asked.

"So you say," I said brutally.

She merely laughed at that. She knew only too well how we all disliked her and disapproved of her slapdash methods on the wards, and the way she bullied the patients in her loud, common voice. She was aware, too, of how the patients hated her but she never let any of it worry her. With her disposition, I suppose she needed a thick skin.

"Well, I can't keep talking to you all night," she said brightly. "I have to meet Hank in half an hour."

"It's a blessing for you that Americans aren't fussy," I said.

"Yes, isn't it?" she said sweetly, making for the door and pausing to look at the photographs on my locker. "Wish you would introduce me to that gorgeous brother of yours though."

"I wouldn't turn you loose on any brother of mine," I said frankly.

She turned at the door and made a face at me. "Cat," she hissed as she went out.

Louise had been giggling to herself all the time that Jean and I had been carrying on the way we usually did. "You are awful, Eve," she said. "But she never gets annoyed no matter what you say to her. In fact, I think she is quite fond of you."

"It pays her to keep on the right side of me, the artful dodger," I said, getting out of bed. "That wretched ward is an absolute shambles every night when I go on duty. I shall report her before I'm through."

"You won't," Louise said comfortably. "You will just carry on, cleaning up for her night after night and letting off steam as you do it. You soon get through it all anyway. Micki's a good kid and the convalescent patients will do more for you in ten minutes than they will for her in a week."

"They would do it for her too if she didn't order them about so," I said crossly. We dressed in shivering silence.

"Louise," I said presently, "do you think a girl could get away with desertion?"

"Physically, yes. Mentally, I doubt it," Louise said serenely.

"But how does one manage about ration books and employment cards?" I asked.

"Oh, there are ways and means. Why? Are you thinking of deserting?"

"Yes, I am," I said defiantly. "I'm sick of this place."

"I thought you seemed to be in a disagreeable mood," Louise said as she creamed her face. "What did dear Cousin Helen have to say?"

"Oh Louise, it's got nothing to do with Helen," I said. "It's all such a waste of time. Where is all this going to get us?"

"Wherever we want it to."

"Oh, it's no use talking to you," I burst out. "You love nursing but I'm sick of it. I hate it—trudging around on burning feet, cleaning wounds and emptying slops."

"Don't tell me you hate nursing," Louise said with a smile.

"But I do," I protested.

"No one who hated it could make as good a job of it as you do," Louise said in her quiet, soothing voice. "The patients all adore you and the doctors and sisters know that they can rely on you for anything."

"That's my natural honesty," I said. "I do this job just as I would do any other, as efficiently as I know how. Any job which I had undertaken in any of the services would have been done in the same way and there would have been a chance of getting promotion—and glory."

Louise burst out laughing. "So it is Cousin Helen," she said. "You shouldn't let her get you down. When she boasts about what she does, you should give her a few details about what goes on here."

"But nothing ever happens here," I pointed out.

"Nonsense. Everything happens here," Louise said as she adjusted her crisp white cap and surveyed the result from all angles. "You could write a book about this place and the people in it."

"But this is only a small emergency hospital," I pointed out. "We don't even get any battle casualties."

"Good heavens! People don't have to be battle casualties to be interesting. We get plenty of air raid casualties and you have some battle casualties on B ward. What about Holt? Then there's Bradley who lost his legs in Crete."

"Yes, I know, but they were patched up before they came here," I said. "The rest of them are just routine surgery and fractures and such."

"So what? They all have their own lives to live, their hopes, ambitions, and personalities, don't they?" Louise answered. "You take stock of them all tonight. Stop looking on them as cases and get to know them." She pulled me down onto the bed beside her and forced me to look at her. "See here, my child," she said. "I'm much older than you are and I know more about life and people than you do. You are in this now and you will be for a long time to come, but don't let it get you down. This war has already dealt you some cruel blows. You don't say much about it and perhaps it would be better for you if you did. But please don't let it embitter you."

Dear, dear Louise, she saw and understood so much. I was lucky indeed to have her as my roommate. No one had seen me cry for a long time, but her kindness was having the worst possible effect. It was only with the greatest difficulty that I managed to keep a firm grip on my emotions.

"I'll try not to," I said, and I really meant it.

"Seriously though, Eve, you should really try to get to know the patients better," Louise went on. "They talk to me quite a lot, you know, no doubt because I am older than all the other nurses. They seem to look on me as a guide, philosopher, and friend. They all like you because of your efficiency and because you do their dressings and treatments with the minimum of fuss."

"Don't be an ass, Louise," I said, feeling very embarrassed. "I do their dressings the way I have been trained, the same as every other nurse does."

"Oh, no. These boys know. You can't fool them," Louise said quickly. "They can tell when anything is being skimped or rushed. They all speak very highly of you, but they say you are always too busy to talk to them. In fact, I don't know if I should say this, but some of them think you are standoffish."

"I don't believe in nurses fraternizing with patients," I said, on the defensive at once.

"There is fraternizing and then there is fraternizing," Louise said with truth. "Take my advice, dear. Come off your high horse and get to know these boys. They're wonderful."

"But if I become too friendly with them they will lose all respect for me," I protested. "Look at Mary Phillipson."

"You would never lose their respect, my dear. As I have said before, these boys are not fools. They know Mary Phillipson for what she is and they know you for what you are."

At that moment Louise was called to the telephone and as I gathered my belongings together for the night I pondered what Louise had said. Was I a snob? Perhaps I was too casual with the patients and inclined to look on them merely as "cases." What had Louise said? "You could write a book about this place." A thought struck me. Why not? I had been trying without success to write fiction since I was twelve years old. Perhaps if I wrote about things around me I would have more success. Many incidents, both touching and amusing, which had happened there, flashed into my mind. I decided that I would jot them down during the rare quiet spells during the night. The more I thought about it the more I liked the idea. If only I could write a book about simple everyday happenings and make it come alive—that would "show" Cousin Helen.

Chapter Three

Louise, Micki, and Diana were already in the dining room when I got there. It was almost half past seven and Barney was spooning out helpings of stiff, gray porridge. There were two letters for me, one from Dorothy and one from Arthur, which I pounced on with glee.

As soon as Barney was out of earshot, Micki and Diana went into details about their afternoon outing. They were both lively, amusing girls and now that I was mentally writing them into my book, I was finding them even more entertaining than usual. In fact, so absorbed had I become with the idea that Barney's strident, "It's ten minutes to eight, you girls. You'd better be off. The day staff has to be relieved sometime you know," did not jar me as it usually did.

Wrapping our capes about us, we gathered up our knitting, writing paper, and bars of chocolate which would help us through the twelve-hour night and set off. It was a beautiful starry night and the brisk walk to the hospital was wonderfully exhilarating.

At the end of the main corridor in the hospital we split up, Louise and Diana to proceed to the two medical wards on the right of the corridor. Micki and I turned a sharp left to the surgical wing—a confusing maze of wards, side wards and private cubicles which accommodated the alarming sum of sixty-eight patients. At the extreme rear were six private rooms for officers, but they were never much bother.

B ward was in confusion as usual when we got there. Sister Hamilton was just scuttling into the duty room, sleeves rolled up and a hypodermic syringe in her hand.

"Good evening, nurses," she said. "It's good to see you. What a day this has been! I have just given Thompson his injection, so if I leave the syringe here perhaps you will be good enough to boil it up for me. I'm sorry the place is in such a mess, but you really can't imagine what it has been like. Higgins had a relapse and had to be rushed to the operating theater at six o'clock. He hasn't been back long so he isn't properly out of the anesthetic yet and Nurse Salter is with him at the moment. I've only had her and Nurse Phillipson on with me since five o'clock, so you can imagine what it has been like. You see, Salter had to be in theater with Higgins all the time and ..."

So it went on. Sister Hamilton was kind and friendly but not efficient enough to run a busy surgical ward. In fairness to her though, no one realized it more than she did. She would have rambled on forever if I had not cut in and tactfully suggested that Nurse Daniels should go along to the officers' section to take the report, so that Nurse Rawley could go off duty.

"Yes, nurse, by all means," Hamilton agreed.

To my relief, Micki was able to disappear. I knew it would not take a minute to get the report from Nurse Rawley and then double back to B ward to start settling the patients down for the night, while I took Hamilton's report and tried to get rid of her as soon as I could. Once she was out of the way, Micki and I would soon get busy, and if things were as quiet on the medical wards as they had been lately, Louise would send Diana down to help us.

First of all, Sister Hamilton took me in to see Higgins. He looked very ill but he was young and had a good constitution. We checked the saline drip which was to continue all night. Nurse Salter was told that she could collect Nurse Phillipson and they could go off duty. We then made a tour of the other beds, while sister rattled off dozens of instructions. Finally I got rid of her and wondered how on earth I would get through all the work before lights out and the duty medical officer's round. I really ought to get Micki to stay with Higgins but I just couldn't spare her.

I went into the day room where a group of noisy convalescent patients was around the fire, smoking, arguing, laughing, reading, and writing. I detailed two of them to make hot drinks for everyone. Two others I put to tidying lockers and emptying ashtrays, and another one I asked to tidy the bathrooms. Webster, recovering from a tonsillectomy, was a trained sick-berth attendant in the Royal Navy, so I told him to sit with Higgins.

Micki appeared at that moment.

"Everything all right up there?" I asked.

"Yes," she replied. "No change, except that Pilot Officer McDonald is due for discharge tomorrow. Commander Taylor is going to make hot drinks for all of them so we don't have to worry about that. How are you getting along?"

"Everything is under control," I said, giving her details and suggesting that we start to tidy the beds.

By nine o'clock the lights were out and all the patients settled down for the night. Shortly afterward the duty medical officer and night sister made their rounds. The officers could keep their lights on for another hour and soon after inspection one of them came down to say there was a pot of tea for us in their kitchen. I sent Micki to have some first and I sat with Higgins. When she came back I thankfully went to have a welcome cup of tea myself.

I was relaxing with a cup of tea and a piece of cake which Commander Taylor had given me when Pilot Officer McDonald came into the kitchen. He was a tall, shy New Zealander who had recently had his appendix removed. I got up to ask what I could do for him but he said he only wanted to let me know that he was being discharged in the morning.

"Oh, yes, I read it in the report," I said. "That's wonderful for you." I poured a cup of tea for him and he sat on the edge of the table.

"I thought I would come in and thank you for everything," he said shyly. "You are always so busy in the mornings. One hardly gets a chance to say anything."

I laughed. "Yes, there is rather a mad rush in the mornings," I agreed.

"Anyway, I think you girls are doing a grand job and I'm so grateful," he said.

"We think you boys are doing a grand job too," I said.

He blushed and there was an awkward pause in which he seemed to be plucking up courage to say something. "Nurse Porter," he suddenly blurted out, "I would like to see you again, that is if you don't think I have a frightful nerve. I-I'm stationed in Kent, you know, and come up to London fairly often but I-I just don't know any girls."

I was about to refuse graciously when I thought of what Louise had said. Was I being standoffish now? Should I get to know the patients better?

"I would like very much to see you again," I said.

"When can I see you?" he asked.

"Well, I shall be on night duty for about six weeks longer, but I get four nights off every two weeks," I said.

"Then I'll keep in touch," he promised. "I never know when I'm going to be flying, but I'm sure we should be able to arrange something soon."

We talked for a few moments longer, then I had to get back to work, so I said goodnight to him and suggested that he should go to bed and get a good night's sleep.

I went out with Mac for the first time about three weeks later, but it was not a very happy evening for either of us. He was so shy and quiet that conversation was stilted and I was tired and jumpy as I always was on my first day off after night duty after trying to adjust to eating and sleeping at normal hours. We had a second-rate dinner and saw a very mediocre film. I think I was mentally comparing him with John. I hated myself for doing this but I just couldn't help it. Supposing John had not been killed, supposing I had been sitting in this cinema with him. In the darkness Mac looked a little like John in his uniform. Oh, how I tried to keep these thoughts from crowding my mind. Mac took me back to the nurses' quarters in a taxi and we said a dismal goodnight. I felt certain that he would never want to see me again, and I didn't care very much either.

The coast was clear, so before going to bed I went along to the hospital and had a cup of tea with Louise. She was in the medical ward kitchen preparing the breakfast trays for the morning and wanted to hear all about my evening out. She was so disappointed when I told her what a dismal evening it had been.

"Did he ask you out again?" she wanted to know.

"Yes, but I think he was just being polite and I don't suppose I shall hear from him again. I'm sure he was just as bored as I was," I said.

"Oh, give the poor boy a break," Louise said quickly. "When a fellow is as shy as he is, you have to give him some encouragement, you know. And Eve, you can be so unapproachable."

It was almost six weeks before I went out with Mac again, but by that time I had spoken to him on the telephone several times, and we had exchanged a few letters. The ice was broken to such an extent that I found myself looking forward to seeing him again. I was, by this time, on day duty again and I met him at Charing Cross station, where he arrived by train at half past seven. We had both eaten dinner so we went to a cinema at Marble Arch.

The main film was almost over when an air raid warning sounded, and as usual, a notice flashed on the screen asking those who wished to leave to do so as quietly as possible and the program would be continued for those who wished to remain. Mac asked me if I wanted to stay, so I said yes and he took my hand in his.

The alert was still on when we left the cinema. Great flashes illuminated the sky, which was filled with the sound of enemy aircraft and the burst of the antiaircraft guns in Hyde Park. We had not realized that the raid was so heavy and for a brief moment we hesitated, then Mac grabbed my arm and we ran along Edgeware Road.

"Mac, we'd better take cover," I said, as the sickening scream of a bomb hurtling through the air seemed all too close. It sounded as though it exploded somewhere near Paddington Station and we ran into the bar of a nearby hotel. It was the first time in my life that I had been in a hotel bar and although I was only there to take cover, I felt terribly guilty about it. There were only about six other people in there, mostly American soldiers, and Mac ordered a beer for himself and a lemonade for me, but we never touched them—I don't know if he even paid for them.

A salvo of bombs fell very close and the building rocked on its foundations. Broken glass fell in all directions and with one accord we all dived under the heavy marble-topped tables and stayed there. The barman put out the dim lights as soon as the windows blew in, but it was still light in there as a full moon shone down and gun flashes dashed madly across the sky.

I knew that I was as close to death as I would ever be, but the awfulness of dying in a pub suddenly struck me. I thought of the minister reading in church the names of church members who had died or who were missing on active service as he did every Sunday before offering prayers for those still serving. I knew that list by heart: Peter Alexander, lost at sea; Larry Armstrong, shot down over Germany; Maurice Floyd, killed in Egypt; Andrew Crossley, missing, believed killed; James Eldridge, missing in Java; Kenneth Farley, taken prisoner at Dunkirk. I could see an addition—Eve Porter, killed in a public bar in London. No one would ever know why I had been there, that I had only sought shelter. They might think that "I had gone to the bad." I felt quite sick.

"Mac," I whispered on a hysterical sob that was almost a laugh. "You'll have to get me out of here. I can't die in a pub. I'm a Methodist." Mac laughed rather shakily as he pressed my left ear to his tunic and placed his hand over my right ear as we huddled there under the table. After what seemed an eternity, the all-clear sounded and we made our way hand-in-hand toward Hyde Park. The park was so breathtakingly lovely bathed in the shimmering silver of moonlight that we sat on a bench to take in its loveliness. It seemed incredible that such a short time before all hell had been let loose in those same skies.

I was supposed to be back in the quarters by midnight, even on a late pass, but time was immaterial. I was still shaking, and it seemed perfectly natural for Mac to place an arm about me and for me to rest my head on his shoulder. How we talked and talked. He told me about his home in New

Zealand, about his parents and his younger brother, his school days, his ambitions, how thrilled his father was because he had been able to visit his relatives in Scotland. I told him about my parents too, my home, my brothers, my job, the Floyds and yes, about John too. He was such an easy person to talk to.

Needless to say, Louise was quite happy about our second date.

My third date with Mac was on his birthday and we had a delightful time. By appointment, we met a crowd of jolly young men from Mac's airfield in the Captain's Cabin, a popular place off Piccadilly. Some of them were members of his own crew. They seemed to be very attached to their captain whom they affectionately called "Cap" and which did not sound much different from the "Mac" I always called him.

They were all New Zealanders with the exception of a navigator called Garth Evans who came from Canada. There was one other pilot, Jack Bluett, who had come with all his crew to celebrate Mac's birthday. Jack was a delightful person and had brought with him a sweet dark-haired girl named Joy Reynolds whom I liked tremendously.

After leaving the Captain's Cabin, we all went along to a night club for dinner and dancing. It was a hilarious evening and what high spirits those boys were in. Looking back now, I marvel at how they managed to remain so cheerful. Most of them were little more than schoolboys, very few of them were old enough to vote. That was Mac's twenty-sixth birthday and he was by far the oldest of all of us, yet these youngsters flirted with death daily. They even joked about it. They sang a macabre song about death, "Here's to the Next Man to Die," but they never admitted that their colleagues had died. They had merely "stopped flying." Maybe that was the only thing to do.

Ah! Happy, carefree youth.

It was not long before Mac and I discovered that we were head over heels in love. How happy we were. What I felt for Mac was so different from what I had felt for John. What I mean is, that by this time I was mature. Thanks to the war and my own experiences, I was far older than my nineteen years. I had adored John throughout my childhood and girlhood years, but now he was gone, leaving me with some very, very happy memories, which, in spite of my love for Mac, I would never want to forget.

Chapter Four

The summer of 1943 was such a happy one for me. There were not many raids over England. We were now on the offensive and hundreds of our planes were droning overhead daily to attack the enemy. Mac was kept busy but we managed to see each other fairly often, sometimes in Kent, but more often in London. Frequently Mac and I with Jack Bluett and Joy Reynolds went out in a foursome. Then in August Jack and Joy were married and Mac was best man. At the same time Mac and I became engaged but we decided that we would not get married until after he came off operations and was safely grounded.

Then, happily, in September Mac and I managed to get leave together. His aunt and uncle had invited both of us to stay with them in Scotland. We traveled on the night train to Edinburgh, a dreary uncomfortable journey at all times during the war, but we were oblivious to everything except each other and the beautiful solitaire diamond which gleamed on the third finger of my left hand.

The journey was continued on another train from Edinburgh, this time not so crowded, and we reached our destination the following afternoon. Mac's aunt met us at the station in an old-fashioned pony and trap. Gasoline by this time was almost a thing of the past for civilians and many old, long unused vehicles were being brought back into service. She drove us through the crisp autumn air to one of the loveliest old houses I have ever stayed in. It was a two-story graystone house with high-raftered ceilings, long windows, and big fireplaces. Mac's aunt, I called her Aunt Margaret from the beginning, showed me to my room, a spacious room with shining mahogany furniture and chintz draperies. There was a huge bay window overlooking the peaceful glen which seemed remote from all the horrors of war. I felt that I must surely be on another planet.

Jeannie, the maid who served tea in the drawing room must have been more than seventy years old, but she moved with the agility of anyone half her age and her black dress and crisp white cap and apron were so very neat. The tea was delicious and the scones were all that one expects Scotch scones to be. I thought there must be at least a month's butter ration spread on them. In fact, there was no noticeable shortage of food at all there. How we stuffed ourselves during the ten days we stayed there.

"Ye need fattening up," old Jeannie said, plying me with food every time I went into her big, spotless kitchen. How those three darlings, Aunt Margaret, Uncle Jamie and Jeannie spoiled us and how we lapped it up. The only son of the house was a missionary in Nigeria and had not been home for five years, so they enjoyed spoiling us.

How I loved the mornings when I could lie in bed late looking out on the peaceful autumn scene, wander downstairs for a leisurely breakfast, and get acquainted with Aunt Margaret and Jeannie. Oh, how we gossiped! Mac and his uncle always went out shooting quite early so we were free to gossip as long as we liked.

During the afternoons Mac and I would go for long walks or Aunt Margaret would take us in the pony and trap to various neighboring houses to show us off and there we would always be stuffed with more delicious food. I was afraid I would not be able to button my uniform when I had to wear it again.

Then, best of all, how I loved those long, lazy evenings when we sat by a huge fire and talked after dinner. Uncle Jamie had a deep resonant voice and so many exciting and hair-raising stories to tell, lots of which we took with a pinch of salt, but it was fun listening to them. About ten o'clock Aunt Margaret would say, "Hold yer blather, Jamie, and let's awae tae bed. The young folks are nae wanting tae listen tae ye all nicht." After they had retired for the night Mac would put out the lights and we would sit in the firelight, the two dogs asleep at our feet. There we talked, planned, dreamed, made love, and forgot the war and the dreadful uncertainty of the future completely.

But, as all good things must end, it was not long before we found ourselves returning south, going back to London and reality, having promised Aunt Margaret we would do our best to get leave over the New Year so that we could go back there and see a real Hogmanay.

Back in London, everyone was asking when the "second front" would be opened up, but no one seemed to have the answer. At the hospital we were as busy as ever.

Gradually autumn passed and winter was with us once more. There were further cuts in food rationing and, oh, how we thanked President Roosevelt for the Lease-lend Act. We became so tired of American spam, dried milk, and powdered eggs but I hate to think how we would have fared without them. No one was really hungry because rationing was fair, but what a dreary, monotonous diet we lived on. Happily for the children, they were well looked after with subsidized milk, orange juice and cod liver oil and in spite of everything, Britain was still producing the bonniest, and in all probability, the healthiest babies in the world.

So we came to another wartime Christmas and, even in wartime, Christmas in British hospitals is always a gay and festive occasion. I joined the hospital choir. We were so lucky that year in having as choirmaster a convalescent patient who in civilian life had been organist and choirmaster at a very big church in Liverpool. After lights out on Christmas Eve, the choir wandered through the wards carrying candles and singing carols. It was so impressive and everyone loved it.

A custom prevalent in British hospitals is for the staff to work round the clock on Christmas Day as it is considered to be the patients' day and I have never heard a doctor or a nurse complain about it. In fact many ask not to be given leave at Christmas as it is often more fun in the hospital than at home and no one likes to miss it. On that one day in the whole year all barriers are broken down. Stiff honorary surgeons, from whom everyone cringes in mortal terror the rest of the year, put on aprons, carve turkeys with professional skill, and wait on junior nurses, but only after the patients have been well and truly stuffed with Christmas fare. Spotless ward floors become covered with gift wrappings, string, boxes and cards, but no one seems to mind a bit.

For weeks before that Christmas of 1943 there seemed to be more expectancy in the air than there had been for some time. Surely, everyone thought, this would be the last Christmas of the war.

Throughout November and December we had a continuous stream of ear, nose, and throat operations—all of them service personnel. One of these cases I remember particularly. His name was Gerald Dudly St. John Ridgeway Travers. He was a tall, painfully thin naval rating of eighteen who came in to have a sinus operation. When he arrived at the hospital, he was a shy reserved youth who seemed almost afraid of his own shadow, but the boisterous influence of the other patients changed him into a vastly different person in a few weeks. For several days he was an "up-patient" whose only treatment consisted of nasal inhalations twice a day. His manners were impeccable. He almost clicked his heels when he came to the treatment room to ask in his cultured voice for his inhalation. The nurses adored him and were quite certain he must be the son of an earl or a duke. Most of the patients, however, were rather dubious about him. I think his Oxford accent gave some of them a complex, so he was something of a lone wolf. If he were around when a nurse was carrying nothing heavier than a hypodermic syringe, he would immediately offer to carry it for her. That alone made some of the patients think him a sissy. However, only two days after his operation, he was sitting up in bed laughing uproariously at the crude jokes of the other three ratings in the same room, and answering good-naturedly to the name of "Charlie." It was not long before he was also making passes at the nurses. I would go in to give him his nasal douche and he would slip an arm about my waist, remarking how tiny it was, and paying many other compliments.

"Now, now, Travers," I would say sternly. "This is not a bit like you. Surely you don't want to get like these other rowdy creatures do you?" I would sweep them all with a withering glance and they would all laugh loudly.

"Of course, he does, nurse. We're educating old Charlie," Bates, the oldest and worldliest of them, would say.

"Yes, and I like it," Travers would say, giving my waist a squeeze. "Do you like it, eh?" and then they would all giggle.

It was often difficult for me to keep a straight face and unfortunately, they knew it, but it really was amusing to see how the boys "educated" Travers. Then, one day, shortly before Christmas, Bates, Travers and four other patients were allowed to go out one afternoon, so they went happily off together.

When I went into their room that night to give Travers his nasal douche, there was a great deal of hilarity in there. I asked if they had enjoyed their outing and they said yes that they had done their Christmas shopping. Then, for some reason or other, they went off into uncontrollable mirth and there was much whispering and nudging. I said they had better quiet down and told Travers to sit down beside his bed so that I could carry out his treatment. He sat down, then politely jumped up and offered to move the chair beneath the light.

"You will be able to see so much better, nurse," he said, with all that old-world charm of his. Unsuspecting, I moved with him beneath the light and someone set the tray down for me. Travers sat down, then immediately jumped up again and took me into a passionate embrace which left me breathless and confused. How they all laughed when I looked up and saw the mistletoe hanging from the light. I pretended to be annoyed, because, understandably, this sort of thing could not be allowed to get out of hand and I threatened to report him. They thought I meant it and pleaded with me to be a sport but I told them with a perfectly straight face that I had to do all in my power to protect young nurses from wolves like Travers. I really put on a good act and sounded very convincing and they were all very subdued right up to the time when I went off duty at eight o'clock that night.

The next morning Sister Hamilton told Travers to report to the Medical Superintendent's office at half past ten, so they were very hostile toward me.

"What a stinking rotten thing to do," Bates said. "You knew it was all in fun."

Of course I repeated all that I had said the night before about maintaining discipline. I knew why Travers had to go to the office, but was not going to say so then. I met him when he was walking along the corridor to the medical superintendent's office. He looked pale and gave me a very dirty look.

Ten minutes later I was in the linen room stacking away clean linen when he burst in wild with excitement. "Nurse Porter!" he gasped. "I'm going home for Christmas. Doc just gave me a pass."

"Yes, I know," was all I said, and then he gave me a big hug and a kiss, but I did not reprimand him this time.

On Christmas morning I received in my mail—in those days, there was still a postal delivery on Christmas Day—a Christmas card on which was written, "To the best little nurse in the world. Love from Charlie," and then, in very tiny writing, "Do you like that, eh?"

Mac had leave for the New Year but I did not, so I insisted that he go to Scotland without me. He had a wonderful time and came back well-fed, relaxed and happy. Then it was back to bombing attacks for him. What a blessing I was kept so busy, otherwise I would have been driven frantic every time I knew that our planes were over enemy territory.

In the spring of 1944 everyone was talking with bated breath about the second front. It was inevitable that it would have to be opened up soon and everyone was impatient for it, especially the troops who had been hanging around for so long and were just itching to get into action.

I managed to get ten days leave in February and went thankfully off to spend it with the Floyds. I was scanning the arrivals and departure boards at Kings Cross Station when I heard someone call my name. I turned and gasped as I beheld Donald Bell.

"Temporary Acting Unpaid Leading Seaman Bell reporting for inspection," he said, grinning his old infectious grin.

Donald had been in the navy now for more than a year but this was the first time I had seen him in uniform. He had always been tall and thin but the uniform made him look about seven feet tall and six inches wide. He had acquired a sailor's typical rolling gait and his hat was pushed back at a rakish angle revealing what he called his "butter-colored" hair. He looked about eighteen years old.

"By the look of you I would say that you liked being in the navy, Donald," I said.

"I would have been born in the navy if I had known what it would be like," he said. He looked quizzically at me and added, "I would say that service life is agreeing with you too," he added. "Tell me, do you do something for that uniform or does it do something for you? Never mind, don't answer. I see you still know how to blush. How's the love life? Reg told me you were engaged. That's wonderful. You see I was right, wasn't I?"

"Yes, you were right," I answered. "What about you? Have you met the girl for you yet?"

"No, not yet," he said with a grin. "Maybe I'm still waiting for you to grow up."

I laughed. "The way you look in that uniform I'd have to wait for you to grow up," I said.

He was coming through London on his way home from embarkation leave and had to rejoin his ship in Chatham that night. He saw me onto my train and talked to me until the train left. He was the same laughing, teasing Donald and I was so glad to see him after such a long time. "If that man of yours doesn't treat you well, just let me know and I'll come and knock his block off," he said as the train pulled out. I hung out of the window and waved until his happy, smiling face was an indistinct blur.

Things were quiet and peaceful those days at the Floyds and I spent ten days of happy relaxation. Noel was overseas again and Dorothy and Al had been married the previous month. It had been a typical, quiet wartime wedding with hardly any friends or relatives free to attend. We were so bitterly disappointed that I could not get the time off to be her bridesmaid, but that was the way it had to be. Mrs. Floyd and Dorothy were of course dying for Mac to come off operational flights so that he and I could be married.

David came to see me. I had written to tell him of my engagement and we were still good friends. "So you are going to leave us to live in New Zealand after the war," he said, looking like a whipped dog.

"Yes," I said, feeling horribly guilty—heaven alone knew why. I had done nothing wrong. Mac was my man and David was not, that's all, but I knew that I would never forget the hurt look in David's kind brown eyes. "Why? Why? Why?" they seemed to say.

Oh! the thrill and suspense of D-day when it finally dawned at last in June of 1944 after those five long, dreary and heartbreaking years. So much has been written about this day in our history and I know that my pen is inadequate to do it, but I can still remember the rumors and speculation which went on as huge convoys of trucks and tanks were making their way southwards through England during those bright summer days prior to D-day. The south of England had become a vast military camp. Once those men involved—British, Australian, New Zealand, African, Canadian, American, Polish, free French and many others—entered the barbed wire enclosures, they were not allowed out again until after the invasion.

The first news of the landings came through on the morning of June 6. I remember sharing a patient's headphones and listening to the account of the first Normandy landings. This was it! The real thing! It was not another Dieppe raid.

That same week the V.1s were launched. At first no one had any idea what they were. I was walking down the hill to the hospital early one morning with a few other nurses when I saw one for the first time. There had been two alerts during the night and we had heard ominous thuds in the distance but thought they were just the usual hit and run raids and that Hitler was having a final fling. As we walked down the hill from the quarters a German plane which appeared to be on fire crashed over some rooftops in the distance. "Oh, look," someone said, "our guns have brought another one down. Hip, hip hooray!"

There were two or three alerts also during the day but nothing out of the ordinary happened, then shortly before midnight the warning sounded again. I was still sharing a room with Louise and she called across to me softly, "Are you awake, Eve?" I said yes and she asked if I wanted to go down to the shelter but I said no I would try to get to sleep again. I turned over but she called out to me again.

"Eve," she said. "You know that plane we saw come down this morning?"

"Yes," I said.

"Well, we didn't shoot it down."

"Of course we shot it down. We saw it didn't we?" I said rather crossly.

"No, it's made like that, with fire in its tail and it's made to come down. It's Hitler's secret weapon," she said.

"What on earth are you talking about?" I asked.

"Well, it's like this. I don't really understand it myself, but this patient who told me about it does. The planes have no pilots in them."

"Good heavens, Louise," I burst out. "How on earth can planes fly without pilots? You must be crazy."

"No, really," she said. "They are launched from the French coast and they fly over here by remote control or something and then, at a certain time, they come down. They are really flying bombs."

"Oh, Louise," I said, still trying to keep up a jocular front. "Someone is pulling your leg, or maybe he has been reading H. G. Wells."

"Eve, it's the truth," she insisted. "The engines shut off and then they fall just as they are intended to."

At that moment we heard one and it seemed to be immediately overhead. The engine had the familiar throbbing sound of the German planes which we had heard so often, but my insides really turned over then. Enemy planes containing pilots had, over the years, become almost commonplace, but enemy planes without pilots—and immediately overhead—were a different matter. As the engine shut off we held our breaths. Was this for us? Suddenly the explosion came but it was further away than we had thought.

During the days that followed more and more became known about the new weapon. V.1s was their official name, but they soon became known by other names—flying bombs, buzz bombs, doodle-bugs and pilotless planes. The *Evening Standard* ran a cartoon one night soon after their launching showing two pilots in a crouching position winging through the air. The caption said simply, "Planeless Pilots." No wonder foreigners think the British mad!

How tired we became during the weeks that followed. The V.Is were the most terrifying weapons we ever experienced. The V.2s which followed later were horrifying but they did not have the same nerve-racking effect on one. The V.2s traveled quicker than sound and, therefore, we neither saw nor heard them coming. They either hit you or they didn't hit you. But the V.1s chug-chugged overhead and those within earshot waited with bated breath, first for the engine to shut off, and then for the crash. Everyone's nerves were worn to a frazzle.

Work in hospitals was, understandably, doubled. Not only were casualties pouring in, but if they came in during the night, as they often did, the night staff could not possibly cope so the day staff had to be roused. If necessary, we were all on call twenty-four hours a day.

Reflecting on all this now, I wonder how we managed to carry on the way we did. We were for the most part, very, very young and needed lots of rest, but we got hardly any. There was additional work, longer hours, the nerve-shattering ordeal of listening for death from the skies and the tragedy of casualties who were coming in at all hours. Many of them were flying glass casualties. Tiny splinters of glass were embedded in limbs, bodies, and eyes. A large number of people had, of course, been buried under their shattered homes and had very extensive injuries.

Most pathetic of all were the children. One can never get used to the idea of children being in the front line of battle. They would cry hour after hour for their mothers and I still cringe when I think of the lies I have told them. "Mummy will be here soon," I would say. "Don't cry any more." I wonder how many children I have damaged psychologically for life because of that lie. Often I knew that at that moment "Mummy" was already dead or that they were still digging for her in the pitiful heap of rubble that had once been a happy home. But what else can one say to a small, weeping, terrified child?

The quarters we occupied were hit by a V.1 just three days after they were first launched. It was shortly before noon. My two-hour off-duty period was almost over and I had to be back at midday. I was standing at the mirror in my bedroom adjusting my cap when it happened. The blast threw me onto Louise's bed and plaster fell like snow from the ceiling. I picked myself up and made my way downstairs to find that it was not as bad as I had thought. Three bedrooms on the south side had been wrecked, as was a storeroom underneath which had not been used for some time. The occupants of the bedrooms were mercifully on duty so there were no casualties. Barney, whom I had half expected to find in hysterics, was completely in command of the situation. I admired her for it, but I thought her "Nurse Porter, aren't you supposed to be back on duty at twelve o'clock?" was uncalled for.

I seemed to be walking ankle deep in glass all the way to the hospital. Not a window was left intact anywhere around and how sorry I felt for a couple of cats I saw picking their way painfully over those tiny fragments of splintered glass.

Both Mac and I were kept so busy during this period that our only means of communication were letters and the telephone, but at the end of July we managed to meet. I had a whole weekend off and went down to Kent. He booked me in at a dear little hotel in the village near the airfield, and although he was on call, we managed to see each other from time to time. Joy was living at the hotel too and had been since she and Jack had been married. She had taken a job as receptionist at the hotel and was thoroughly enjoying it. Having had asthma all her life, Joy did not have to go into the services and could, within reason, pick and choose her jobs.

On that Saturday night Joy and I had dinner at the airfield with Mac and Jack and then on Sunday morning we were all going to church together. However, at the last moment, Mac could not go, so the three of us went. He did, however, manage to take me to the station when I left on Sunday night. It was a glorious sunny evening and we were so aware of the deliciousness of English summer evenings—the happy birdsong, the hum of lawnmowers, and the smell of newly-cut grass—as we made our way to the railway station.

"Do take care of yourself, darling," Mac said as he put me on the train.

"You practice what you preach, my lad," I said with a bantering note. "Don't forget that I want you all to myself and in one piece when the war is over."

"It can't be long now," he said. "Not many more months surely, then it's off to New Zealand for us."

I hung out of the carriage window and watched him for as long as I could after the train pulled out of the station. He looked so boyish and handsome, yet I had noticed lines on his face which had not been there the last time I had seen him. He looked tired too. It was difficult to pinpoint but he really was beginning to show the strain of it all. I wished with all my heart that they would take him off operations if only for a short spell. I worried about him every moment that I was away from him and I knew that he was just as worried about me. We were both feeling the strain of war and work and anxiety to the same extent. Would we ever feel young and carefree again? It was a big question.

At the end of that week I received a letter from Joy. It had come by the afternoon post and Jean Harris brought it to me on the ward. I wondered what Joy could be writing to me about but did not have time to open it then as I was about to go into the operating theater with a patient, so I slipped it in my pocket. I remembered it again after the operation was over and I was sitting beside the patient's bed waiting for him to regain consciousness. The operation, although interesting, had seemed pointless. Mr. Douglass was a very tired cantankerous old man and everyone knew that his cancer was too deep-seated for surgery to do much good.

"I don't know how to begin this letter," Joy wrote. "But, as Jack says, who else is there to let you know? You must be brave, my dear. My heart and soul are with you." I knew without reading any further what was coming, but I read on mechanically. There was no hope that he had been taken prisoner. Jack had seen Mac's plane go down in flames. Mac had "stopped flying."

What does a nurse do when she receives such news on duty?

Well, she keeps a stiff upper lip and carries on. She must not show her private emotions. She is not supposed to have any. Mr. Douglass opened his eyes and asked for a drink. I quietly told him he could not have anything to drink yet, but I moistened his lips. He dropped off for a while and then he rallied and started throwing himself about.

"There, there Mr. Douglass," I said. "Just try to lie quietly. It's all over and you are back in your own bed." Then he vomited, very noisily and very messily.

Diana Bourne, hearing him, came to my rescue. "Oh, the poor old thing," she said compassionately. "Here, let me give you a hand."

"Stay with him a moment, will you," I said. "I'll just empty this bowl and get some clean sheets and towels, then we can clean him up. Shan't be long."

I had just cleaned the bowl and was on my way to get the clean linen when it happened—a direct hit on the hospital. I threw myself flat on the floor as I felt the earth shake beneath me and plaster falling all over me. As soon as I could, I got up and brushed myself down with trembling hands. As in a daze I made my way back to Mr. Douglass' room. The outer wall was completely demolished and Diana was lying face down beneath the debris. Other people were coming from all directions now but I was only vaguely aware of it as I tore with my bare hands at the bricks and mortar in a desperate effort to release Diana, but she had been killed instantly. Diana—vital, laughing, lively, eighteen-year-old little Diana—had died in that split second when I had been out of the room. Mac—my darling Mac—was dead too, and over in his bed in the corner, Mr. Douglass, old, crotchety and riddled with cancer, lived on.

For the first time in my life I forgot the dignity of the profession and behaved as no nurse should ever behave. I had reached the end of my tether and broke into uncontrollable sobbing. Never will I forget the kindness of everyone during the weeks that followed. The matron insisted on sending me home for a good rest.

"No one needs a rest more than you do, my dear," she said kindly. "Then, if you think a change of hospital would benefit you I won't object to a transfer. I would be very sorry to lose you, you know that, but if it would help, don't hesitate to tell me."

The Floyds were as kind to me as ever and so was dear, devoted David.

While I was on leave I went to see Mrs. Duncan, my commandant and we had a long, long talk together. It was she who suggested that I might like to apply for an overseas posting. "It might be the very thing for you at the present time," she said, "and as your matron is willing for you to be transferred, I can make the suggestion without any qualms." So that was how I came to make application for overseas service.

I was back at the hospital when headquarters notified me that I was being considered for an overseas posting. I began to visualize what it would be like and wondered where I would be sent. I found myself looking forward to the outcome and thought that I might even eventually march into Berlin itself with the glorious British Liberation Army. The far east did not enter my head so it was with something of a shock that I received a letter from headquarters asking me if I would be willing to go to India. Something else which had never entered my head was to say no to a commanding officer, so I said yes, I would go to India.

Chapter Five

When called upon, I duly attended a selection board at Headquarters and was accepted. I was thrilled to find Lady Mountbatten on the board as she was the head of all V.A.D. personnel in India and South East Asia Command. Soon after that, things really began to happen. The next few weeks were hectic with visits to headquarters and the India office, signing papers, having medical examinations, drawing tropical kit allowance, having injections, attending lectures on tropical diseases and life in the tropics, scouring London for a metal trunk. Metal trunks all seemed to have gone underground, but I found out later that there was a basement full of them at headquarters which I could have had for far less money than I eventually paid for one, but that was one of the things they forgot to tell me.

Finally all was ready. My purchases were completed, goodbyes had been said, my will drawn up and my metal trunk tied to a taxi. I was on my way to the transit camp where I would at last be able to see what my traveling companions were like. My contract for this assignment was for two years or the duration of the war, whichever proved to be earlier.

We were accommodated reasonably comfortably at an army hostel for two days. There we got to know each other and sorted ourselves into pairs and groups the way a crowd of human beings always will. I found myself sleeping in a dormitory that had eighteen beds in it and what an assorted group we were. Lying in bed listening to all the different dialects was an entertainment in itself. There were girls with lilting Scottish accents, one from Wales, two from Devonshire, one from Tyneside, several from Lancashire, and others with their clipped BBC voices might have come from any part of the British Isles.

Many of the girls it seemed, especially those from small towns and villages, had not purchased all their equipment. They were hoping to find time to complete their shopping in London. As things turned out they had lots of time.

Those two days were filled to capacity. In between dashing here, there, and everywhere, we had to attend numerous roll calls, sometimes at headquarters, sometimes at the transit camp, but we never seemed to get any nearer to finding out just when we would be leaving, or the port of embarkation. But at last the big moment arrived. A whispering, excited mob assembled in the lounge to await the arrival of an important man from the India office who was to tell us, at last, the port and the time of our departure. It was all very hush-hush of course.

Never will I forget the tense drama of his arrival. There was a breathless hush and one could almost hear everyone's inside turn a somersault. A highly-strung Scots lass next to me gripped me by the arm and said between clenched teeth, "I canna stand it." Actually her emotion was being wasted. All he said was that there was a hold up at the docks and we would be given railway warrants to our home towns. We were to report back in ten days' time unless we heard anything to the contrary in the meantime.

Things seemed very flat after that, so we made arrangements about our trunks and began to peruse timetables. I decided to travel north on the 10:15 that night with another girl who was going to Darlington on the same train. She told me she had found a wonderful eating house where you could get eggs—the old-fashioned kind that came out of shells—and real steaks to eat. She was positively drooling as she told me and so was I. I agreed to go with her for a meal but told her that I refused to believe her until I actually saw the steak and eggs in front of me.

As it turned out she was right. It was a funny little place somewhere off Fleet Street. There were marble-topped tables and very little in the way of interior decoration, but what they lacked in comfort, they made up for in the prewar luxury of the food. How we enjoyed both the food and the company.

There were journalists, taxi drivers, a sprinkling of Americans and crowds of lively Australians there.

The journey north was agreeable enough. We shared a compartment with two naval officers, an American army nurse and a dried-up elderly civilian. From the station I took a taxi to the Floyds and rapped loudly on the door to awaken them. It was not quite half past six in the morning. Mrs. Floyd almost fell out of the window when she looked out to see who it was.

"Good gracious," she gasped. "I thought you would be on the high seas now."

"So did I," I said bitterly.

After ten days I again found myself among my colleagues at the transit camp and although our previous acquaintance had been of such short duration, we greeted each other like long lost relatives. The India office did not waste any more time and the next morning, bright and early, we lined up in the hall and, in a very orderly manner, were marched to waiting trucks which took us to the military station at Addison Road. We were actually at the station before we were told that our port of embarkation was Southampton, but we still did not know the name of the ship. We were on board when we found that out.

On the train I shared a compartment with two Canadian girls, Elizabeth Arthur and Mildred James, and it was the beginning of a very happy friendship. Mildred was an attractive girl and Elizabeth, with prematurely gray hair and flawless complexion, was really striking. They told me they had been nursing in England for a year and had the option of either returning to Canada or signing up for service in India. I admired them for choosing the latter because it meant they had to drop to British rates of pay and I believe that our rules and regulations were much more rigid than theirs.

At Southampton I had a strange sinking feeling as I stepped off England onto a gangway. Would I ever return, I wondered? I was vaguely aware of hundreds of troops who were already on board leaning over the rails and cheering as we filed on board.

I found myself in a cabin on the promenade deck, which by some expert planning, they had managed to squeeze in thirteen bunks, in two and three tiers. I have no doubt that for peacetime traveling it had been a four berth cabin but for transporting service personnel all luxuries such as dressing tables and wardrobes were removed to be replaced by bunks.

The draft conducting officer told us that we had time to write letters before we sailed. He also said that as we had officer status, we could censor our own mail, but that we were honor bound not to mention the name of the ship or the port. We swelled with pride to think that the army was putting so much trust in us, but it was not until some time later that we found out that the army was not really taking any chance on our honor. Those letters did not leave Southampton until five days after the ship sailed.

Within three hours of embarking, the ship pulled out. There was nothing spectacular about it—no crowds, no streamers and no hidden band bursting into "Rule Britannia." By straining very hard I managed to count five workmen on the dockside, so I waved hopefully. This was the first time I had said good-bye to England and it was hard trying to keep down a lump which would keep rising in my throat. A tall girl standing beside me said, "Thank goodness I have caught up with my father at last. He has been to India five times and now this is my fifth." I felt like a very inexperienced and unsophisticated traveler.

The trip was very pleasant and full of interest. There were almost two thousand men on board and only eighty women. A quickly formed entertainment committee arranged dances, films, sports and concerts. A dashing young army officer gave lectures on Urdu which were well attended at first but the novelty soon wore off.

The two Canadian nurses and I spent a lot of time on the boat deck with a crowd of men who had been to India before. They told us many amusing stories of their adventures there too.

Often when lounging on deck we forced ourselves to read an alarming little book which had been issued by the India office. It was called "Hints on Health in India" and went into morbid details about the horrible diseases one might get in India. We had attended lectures on tropical diseases in London of course but they had dealt mainly with malaria, dysentery, beriberi and dengue fever, but it seemed that more than half the terrors of life in the tropics had been withheld. Why, an innocent act like brushing one's teeth with the water on a train could result in violent death from cholera, and if one took so much as one step barefooted, thousands of hookworms would immediately work their way from the soles of the feet to the intestines.

In addition, apparently there were some unpleasant little microbes which, without the slightest encouragement would lay eggs in ears and noses. Others would make for abrasions in the skin and burrow happily through the tissues for years. In fact, there seemed to be no limit to the dangers which lurked everywhere for the unsuspecting European. How anyone could possibly avoid so many diseases was beyond all belief, and even if one could dodge them there was always the chance of being bitten by a mad dog or a poisonous snake.

"Gee, it looks like this is going to be a one-way trip for most of us," Mildred would say looking up from her book in alarm. We had visions of the rare viruses in India already passing the word around that we were on our way and arranging a mass attack as soon as we stepped off the ship—something like Hitler's Fifth Column. I doubt if we had ever felt nearer to certain death even in the blitz. The only comfort we had was that the men on board who had been to India previously looked quite healthy and did not seem unduly perturbed about going back there.

Mildred and I were usually to be found with the same four men, all Royal Engineers. Bill was a big, quick-witted fellow from Liverpool, and Arthur, a very shy reserved youth with, I was certain, little or no experience with women. The other two, Philip and Eric were born comedians.

As the nights grew hotter and hotter we were usually to be found in the same spot on the promenade deck drinking glass after glass of cold drinks and listening to the boys' highly amusing tales of their experiences in India. Many of their tales we took with a pinch of salt, but they made good listening.

Elizabeth we saw very little of during the evenings as she had unfortunately fallen in love with one of the ship's officers. I warned her that shipboard romances should never be taken seriously and that any man on board ship automatically attains a certain amount of glamour, but it was all to no avail. I was to find out later that Elizabeth had a disconcerting habit of falling in love misguidedly and often.

So the days slipped happily and lazily by. Our spells of ship's hospital duty were few and far between as there was very little sickness on board and nothing serious. All too soon Bill came to find me one morning to tell me that Bombay was in sight. I went up on deck and stood beside him at the rail with a strange feeling of sadness and excite-

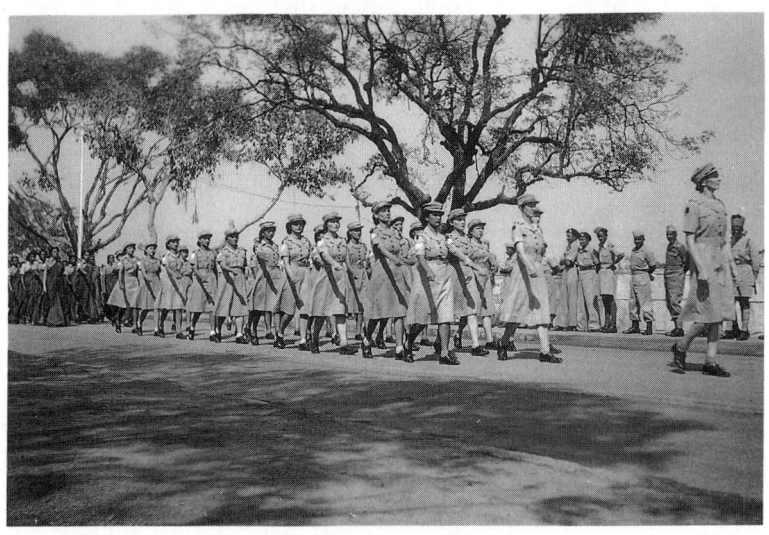

British and Indian Servicewomen

ment inside me. As Bombay drew nearer he was able to point out various landmarks to me and promised that if we were allowed ashore before finally dispersing he would take me to all the places of interest.

We tied up at Alexandra Dock and found ourselves immediately opposite the post office where the mail was being sorted on the ground outside. The dockside was terribly dirty and had a characteristic odor. Bill said it was India that I could smell and that I would not even notice it after a while. He told me to look closely at the mail sorters and to marvel at the fact that mail ever reached its destination at all. They were squatting on the ground and sorting the mail into various bundles. Then they were resorting the bundles and so far as I could make out were putting them on the same piles again. Bill assured me that none of them could read or write.

A group of natives was squatting on the dock side gazing unemotionally at the scene around, occasionally scratching themselves and spitting. It really was a fascinating scene for me. An elderly man wearing a loincloth, a dirty turban and a long off-white beard was working a crane immediately above us. His speed, like that of the mail sorters, was almost dead slow. A few beautiful Anglo-Indian members of the Women's Royal Naval Service kept appearing on the scene from somewhere and then disappearing again. We watched various people coming aboard and as two white women in smart tropical kit walked up the gangway I marveled at their healthy appearance. They certainly did not look as though they had been "got at" by microbes yet, and I took heart.

Elizabeth came up in great excitement. Her boyfriend had been ashore and bought her a hand of bananas, which she was distributing generously. I took one and gazed at it in awe. "Elizabeth," I said reverently, "do you realize that it's been almost five years since I saw a banana?"

Arthur appeared just as I was about to relieve my banana of its skin and told me to make sure that the skin was undamaged and not to eat the ends. It rather spoilt my enjoyment as I could see that a simple pleasure like eating a banana was fraught with danger.

We did not officially disembark until two days after the ship docked but the following day we were allowed ashore from ten o'clock in the morning until half past eleven at night. Bill, Philip, and Eric went ashore early to make arrangements about rejoining their units and Mildred and I went later with Arthur. I was amazed to find the streets so wide and straight and gasped in ecstasy when I saw the wonderful goods displayed in the shops, things which had not been seen in Britain for years. The pavements I noticed were covered with red splashes. "That isn't blood," Arthur hastened to assure me. "It's betel nut juice. These people chew it all the time and spit all over the place, so be careful when you walk below upper stories."

It was not far to our rendezvous with Bill and the two boys, so we walked. It was incredibly hot and I hoped that I would be able to stand up to the heat. Actually, it never had any effect on me all of the time I was in India. In fact, I seemed to thrive on it. We had a snack when we met the boys, first making sure that we found a cafe that was "in bounds to British troops." I ate my first snack in India with very mixed feelings, wondering if I had already sown the first seeds of cholera or typhoid.

Later we all went for a trip around Marine Drive in a gharry, a type of cab peculiar to Bombay, drawn by an ancient horse, alighting at various places of interest enroute and to count the bug bites which we had already acquired in the gharry. The boys proved to be most interesting guides and their knowledge of the currency and language was a great help.

Around one o'clock we found ourselves near the Gateway to India so we dismissed the gharry and went to lunch at a nearby Chinese restaurant which the boys knew and recommended. The party split up after lunch. Philip and Eric went to look up some fellow officers who were stationed at Malabar, while Mildred and Arthur went to Beach Candy, and Bill asked me if I would like to go with him to visit some friends who lived in a block of flats near the Taj Mahal Hotel. Unfortunately when we got there we found they were on leave in the hills, so we went shopping. First we visited the elite emporiums on Hornby Road, but later we went to the more obscure but highly entertaining shops off the beaten track. Bill wanted to buy me everything I liked until I was almost afraid to admire anything. The narrow, dirty streets I found packed with action, but the stench was increasingly nauseating. There was a delightful half hour in the shop of an elderly Parsee gentleman who invited us inside to shelter from a sudden and heavy shower of rain. The monsoon season was not quite over and I discovered that out of a cloudless blue sky, a shower of tropical rain could swoop down without warning and drench one in a matter of seconds. The sudden reappearance of the sun though dried one almost as quickly.

We dined fairly early at the Taj Mahal Hotel and then went to a cinema which I was amazed to find was the last word in luxury. An Andy Hardy film was showing and the audience was composed mainly of Indians who laughed hysterically throughout the entire film. I did not think it as funny as all that.

We rounded off the day by having supper at the Taj and joined the dancers, where we saw several of our fellow passengers including Arthur and Mildred.

All too soon, it seemed, we had to make our way back to the ship. There had been another shower and the streets seemed fresh and cool. I noticed natives sleeping soundly on doorsteps, on the pavements and even in the middle of the roadway. The gharry had to make several swerves to avoid running over them. Bill assured me I would soon get used to that sort of thing—Indians could sleep anywhere at any time.

There was as much activity on the dock and on the ship when we got back as there had been during the day. We stood on deck for quite a long time watching the noisy chattering group of coolies unloading, and talking about the wonderful time we had had that day and throughout the trip. Naturally I was wondering what I would be doing twenty-four hours from then. We knew by then that all the nursing staff on the ship was leaving for Poona first thing in the morning.

Chapter Six

It was quite touching the following morning watching the troops disembark. Everything was carried out with remarkable efficiency. The various regiments were assembled and marched off the ship, where, between mountains of luggage and mail bags, they formed into groups of threes and were marched to waiting trains. Officers and noncommissioned officers who were familiar to the country were put in charge of troops going in various directions. Bill was one of the first to leave; it was six o'clock and he was taking about forty men to Jhansi. I watched him assemble them and march them off and out of sight. Poor boys, they looked so young and so very hot with their heavy kit bags and paraphernalia which the war office insisted they must carry personally.

It was almost eight o'clock when we disembarked and Arthur, Philip, and Eric were still on board. We kept waving to them as we walked away from the dock. They looked so small from there and soon they were out of sight altogether.

The acute discomfort to be experienced on Indian trains had frequently figured in the boys' conversations with us, but our trip to Poona was all that could be desired. The army must have been trying to create an impression by putting a hospital train at the disposal of the newly arrived Queen Alexandra's Imperial Military Nursing Service and Voluntary Aid Detachment personnel.

We spread ourselves out on the comfortable berths and prepared to enjoy the comparatively short journey. There was a constant stream of Indian army boys passing through the compartments with food, drinks, fruit, books, and magazines. At the stations where we stopped enroute, small beggar boys entertained us by singing and clamored for *baksheesh*, grinning all over their little brown faces.

Poona was vastly different from Bombay although it was not such a good shopping center and our quarters were not the best. However, we soon adapted ourselves to the life there. The hospital compound was very fresh and green after the monsoons, and the wards were pleasant. It was strange having so many insects about at first, but gradually we got used to them and soon learned even to identify them. Sleeping under a mosquito net was a novelty too.

Unfortunately, in those days I did not keep a diary although I intended to and so far as Poona is concerned my memory is rather hazy. Actually I never really cared for the place. The famous Poona Club was set in beautiful surroundings but the atmosphere was rather that of an elderly gentlemen's club in St. James. It may have been the "Mecca of the Pukka" but it was not for me.

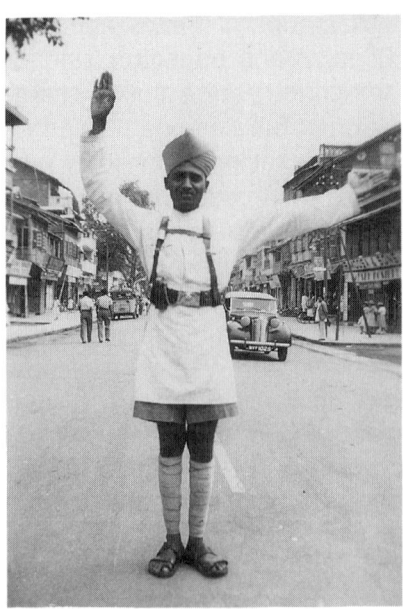
Traffic Officer, Main Street, Poona

The majority of the girls whom I had become acquainted with on board ship were sent to various parts of India but, happily for us, Elizabeth, Mildred and I were at the same hospital in Poona for some time. Elizabeth and I were on the same ward. It was officers' TB (tuberculosis) ward and we found it terribly depressing as the patients were so young and the disease, in most cases, so deep-rooted. Most of them were victims of the heat and damp of the jungle.

India was a hopeless place in which to nurse TB patients. One boy I remember in particular was a major—ridiculously young to be a major, but that is the way it was during the war. His name was Morgan and his home was in North Wales.

Elizabeth, having visited Wales a few months previously was able to converse with him about many places there. He had fits of acute depression, but Elizabeth usually managed to get him out of them.

Off duty there was much to take our minds off the depression of the ward. There were many parties at the club and in numerous messes. Sometimes we went to the British Other Ranks' (B.O.R.) dances. We felt it our duty since the poor, unfortunate B.O.R.s seldom had the chance of meeting white girls, and even then, the chance of getting to dance with one was very remote as there were usually about thirty men to one white girl. For most of them their only chance of dancing with a girl was in the "excuse me" dances. They congregated in a solid mass in the middle of the floor while the more fortunate males with partners danced around them. They were not allowed to excuse a couple until the emcee blew his whistle, then it was every man for himself. It became quite commonplace to see men dancing together and some of them danced very well together, too.

When we were off duty together in the afternoons, Elizabeth and I often met two convalescent officers at Murratore's for tea. One of them came from Elizabeth's hometown in Nova Scotia and the other from my hometown in Yorkshire. We could never quite get over the coincidence of it.

It amuses me now to think of the way in which, during the first few weeks in the mess, we religiously covered butter dishes, sugar bowls and jam pots immediately after we had extracted what we wanted, but after we got used to the sight of ants crawling all over our food, we were not quite so fussy.

"Always shake your shoes before putting them on and always turn down your bed before getting into it," we were told over and over again, and I am afraid I had to learn the hard way about shaking my shoes. One morning, forgetting about it completely, I quickly put on a shoe and a killer scorpion ran out of the toe to make room for my foot. What a blessing the shoe had an open toe! Needless to say I was never careless about that again. Then, one night, one of the nurses forgot to turn down her sheet and as she pushed her feet down, she touched a snake which was curled up at the foot of the bed. How quickly she leaped out and how she screamed! Another girl in a deep sleep, had her elbow eaten to the bone by a rat before she woke up. Then there was the occasion when I came into my bungalow one night and switched on the light. The fan switch was also beside the door and I was about to switch that on too when I looked up and saw a python curled around the stem of the fan. It had come in through the roof and I shot out through the door yelling for the guard to come and shoot it.

Tucking the mosquito nets tightly around our beds at sundown and then crawling underneath them when we finally went to bed was another ritual that went by the board.

So the time went by. Within two months I felt that I had been in India for years and was, I regret to say, very condescending to more recent arrivals. It was not long before poor Elizabeth realized that her idol on the ship had feet of clay. But in between telling me how heartbroken she was, she was managing to find plenty of consolation.

Bill wrote regularly and asked me to try and get a posting to Jhansi. I promised to apply for a transfer but somehow never got around to it. Christmas and New Year's passed. They were very strange and unnatural in the heat of the tropics. I asked Bill in a letter what kind of Christmas he had spent. He wrote back and said that he had been to Calcutta on a special mission and had driven there and back. His Christmas dinner was a tin of corned beef by the roadside. He sounded very fed up and asked if I would please spend a leave with him in Mussoorie. He said I would love the place and we would have a wonderful program of skiing and tobogganing. It sounded very attractive and I said I would love it as soon as I was eligible for a twenty-eight day leave.

And then the war in Europe was over. With alarming, destructive, and breathtaking suddenness the world entered the Atomic Age and the war was over. Over! It was hard to predict what would happen in the Far East so we just carried on with our work and hoped for the best. There was no thought then of dropping atom bombs but it was a great comfort to know that no more bombs would be dropped on England.

The next monsoon season found the three of us in Kalyan and it was awful. The quarters were worse than they had been in Poona and everything was damp and musty. Mildred had a nasty fall in a monsoon trench and was in bed for three weeks. The population in Kalyan changed too often for Elizabeth to get any ideas about them.

Mildred was a vastly different person from Elizabeth. She was older than we were—I think she was about thirty—and thought all our male acquaintances "sweet kids." I rather think that she herself had ideas about a "sweet kid" whom she wrote to in the British Liberation Army. She always waxed sentimental when she got a letter from him, but it never came to anything.

Bearers in Kalyan were few and far between and we thought ourselves lucky to have one between the three of us. Actually he was about as much use as a sick headache, but he was such an engaging creature and the way he woke us up in the mornings was worth the money. His voice, so soft and musical, would call very, very gently and he would go on calling without raising his voice a fraction for however long we took to wake. I would sometimes deliberately pretend to go on sleeping just to see if he would raise his voice, but he never did. Then I would open my eyes slowly and say, "Good morning, Ali." The most beautiful smile would break out on his finely chiseled features as he said pleasantly, "Good morning, Sister sahib. *Char monkter?*" And he would hold out a cup of lukewarm tea with far too much sugar in it.

Great preparations had been made all over India to receive our prisoners of war from Japanese camps, but, once they were liberated, morale was so high among them that thousands were found fit to travel back to England far sooner than had been expected. Consequently many hospitals began to close. The magic word on everyone's lips now was "demobilization" and all began to work out their "group numbers."

A letter from Bill informed me that he had been transferred to Delhi, "among the brass hats." He said Delhi was a beautiful city and that I would love it. He wanted me to try to get a transfer there and he said he would see that I had a wonderful time. But by that time I was already on the move again myself. Even the nurses were never kept long in Kalyan. The climate was cruel and there was pathetically little in the way of relaxation.

Elizabeth, Mildred, and I were still together and we were all three going to the 75 General Hospital which was somewhere near Ranchi in Bihar State. Two other girls, Jill Norman and Fay Harrison, were traveling in the same direction. They were going to the Combined Military Hospital in Ranchi.

The monsoon season was almost over when we left for Calcutta, the first jumping off stage on our journey. We joined a troop train at Kalyan which had come up from Bombay and Elizabeth and I went into a compartment with two other nurses who had come up from Bombay. They had some army officer friends on the same train who came along at intervals during the next two days to play cards. It was so hot and sticky traveling, and at every station we were pestered by dirty, smelly beggars.

Mildred, being the oldest, was in charge of our party, and every time the train stopped, she dashed along the platform like a broody hen to make sure that we were still there. Very few trains in India have corridors so communications with people in other compartments had to be when the trains were standing in stations. The first night on the train Elizabeth and I had just climbed to our upper berths and were settling down for the night when she let out a strangled yelp. A previous occupant had scribbled a lewd picture immediately above her head. She said she objected to having to look at it all night so I suggested that she put the light out and shut up.

Chapter Seven

Calcutta seemed even hotter than Kalyan. We just steamed. On leaving the train, Elizabeth, Jill, and I sat on our trunks while Mildred and Fay went to the railway traffic officer's (R.T.O.) office to make reservations for the remainder of the journey. Suburban trains were discharging shop and office workers by the thousands. It was fun watching them. Some wore European clothes, others part-European and part-Indian. All wore European shirts with the tails outside their trousers or *dhotis* and the majority wore shoes but no socks.

After what seemed an eternity, Mildred and Fay returned accompanied by a fussy little Indian captain, who explained that he was the R.T.O. and that he could not guarantee reservations to Ranchi for at least two days, but that he would escort us personally to the Grand Hotel and arrange accommodation for us. He was a very kind and sincere little man. We were almost sorry when he left us. We and our twenty-one pieces of luggage were piled into a truck and off we set, the little captain keeping up a constant flow of conversation from his perch beside the driver. At the Grand Hotel a small army of coolies transferred our goods and chattels to the lobby and the little captain went to the desk to make reservations for us. The Grand Hotel, at that time, was for British and American officers only and had its own resident R.T.O., a British major. There were hundreds of male officers staying there but hardly any women, so we were stared at by all.

We saw a nursing sister there whom we had known in Poona. She was alone, so she pounced upon us with glee. "I've been here two days waiting for a reservation to Dacca," she said. "My husband is there and I have managed to get a transfer there. Isn't it wonderful?" We agreed that she was indeed lucky as it seemed to be army policy to keep husbands and wives as far away from each other as possible. It transpired that she had two empty beds in her room, so Jill and Fay arranged to occupy them.

Elizabeth, Mildred, and I were allotted a fairly decent room for three. It had three clean and very comfortable beds, lots of space, a screened balcony and a bathroom. Having plumbing and sanitation was an unheard-of luxury for us. How we appreciated it.

As soon as we could, we ejected the large chattering crowd of coolies, porters, hangers-on, and of course the still voluble captain from the room. Then stripping off our travel-stained khaki drill, we made for the bathroom—we had not seen a real bathtub since Poona. However, we found an elderly sweeper sound asleep on the bathroom floor, so he had to be roused and thrown out.

Immediately when we appeared in the lounge of the hotel, we were inundated with offers of dates, but Elizabeth espied a lonely figure whom we knew sitting in a basket chair beneath a fan. He was a Royal Worcestershire Regiment major who had come over on the same ship as we had and his rather dejected appearance brightened considerably when we hailed him. He jumped up and almost shook our hands off and said how glad he was to see us. He said that we could have celebrated our reunion but unfortunately he was leaving for Delhi that day. He was recently back from Burma and had been in Calcutta for five days feeling thoroughly fed up.

"Now, on my last day, I meet you lovely creatures," he moaned.

Thinking that it would cheer him up to be seen around town in the company of five white women, we asked him to show us around. It was a rare sight in India to see one man surrounded by several British women, it was usually the reverse. Len became the focus of many envious glances from the crowds of Britons and Americans.

"I haven't spoken to a white woman for more than six months," Len said, "and now I'm surrounded. The trouble is if I tell anyone they'll never believe me."

We went into the Great Eastern Hotel for lunch and again were the only white women among a crowd of American officers. "Gee, brother, what do you have?" they asked Len as he passed.

At the table I took a long drink of water but almost spat it out. There had recently been an outbreak of cholera in Calcutta, so now everything was so highly chlorinated it was nauseating.

Before dinner that night we went to the station to see Len off. He found himself very popular among his fellow travelers and then, among the crowds of people on the platform, we spotted our dear little R.T.O. friend of the morning. He bounded over to us and shook us all by the hand, including Len and asked if we wanted a lift back to the hotel. He was going there very shortly with a party which had just arrived.

We accepted gratefully, and after Len's train had pulled out, the little captain took us to a waiting coach which contained about fifteen Americans, six of whom were going to the Grand Hotel. They were a lively crowd of fellows, also just back from Burma, and when they heard that we too were staying at the Grand, they suggested that we form a party and go to the Coconut Grove. We enjoyed ourselves tremendously there, although my partner, a young lieutenant from Texas, was a very poor dancer and a man of few words.

They all left Calcutta the next day and it looked as though we would have to remain there over the weekend. However, it turned out to be most entertaining, as we teamed up with a crowd of British army officers who were awaiting transportation to Saigon. I was partnered by a handsome Scot who had been in the army in India for close to ten years. He was very witty and an excellent dancer and he knew Calcutta like his own backyard. What an excellent guide he was too.

It was very amusing one night when Keith was buying a corsage for me from a curbside seller. A very small boy kept pestering him and Keith answered him in Urdu. As we waited for a taxi the boy still hung around us. "What is he saying, Keith?" I asked repeatedly and finally he told me.

"He wants to know if I want a woman," Keith said, angrily.

"Well, what on earth does he think I am?" I asked indignantly.

Keith threw back his head and laughed heartily, then he looked down at me, with his blue eyes twinkling. "Oh, my sweet innocent child," he said. "It isn't quite the same thing." I blushed and was horrified that such a small boy should be soliciting prostitution.

At Keith's laughter the boy pestered him yet again, so Keith turned on him angrily. "No—I don't want a woman," he roared.

The boy, quick as lightning, came in again. "Well, you want boy then, sahib?" he asked with a lewd grin. Luckily at that moment we got a taxi.

What a delightful time we had during those few days in Calcutta. We had delicious meals at Firpo's and went dancing

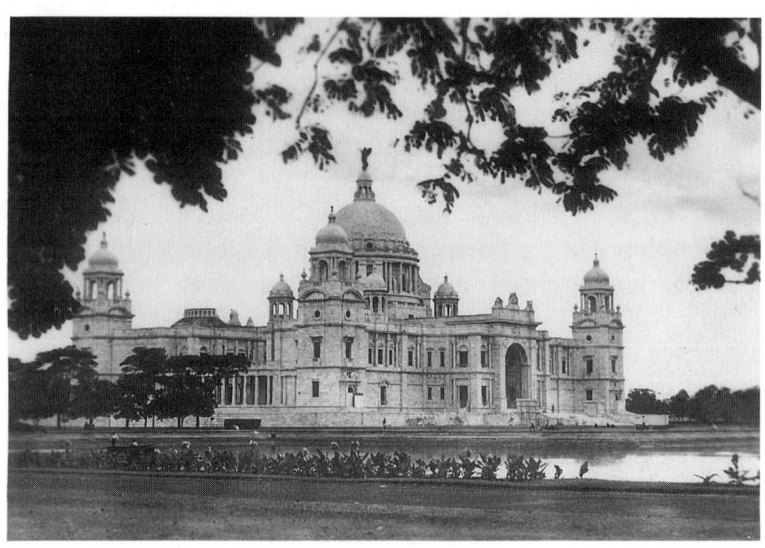

Victoria Memorial, Calcutta

at the various clubs and hotels. We saw all the sights of Calcutta and in the heat of the afternoons we sat in air-conditioned cinemas. Sometimes we sat in the palm court of the Grand Hotel and listened to the hotel orchestra. Their favorite tune seemed to be "I'll Be Seeing You," which they played over and over again. I never hear that tune now without being wafted back there on waves of memory.

It was on the following Tuesday morning that we paid our daily visit to the R.T.O.'s office in the hotel and learned that reservations had been made for our party. We were to entrain that evening at half past five and our escorts, it seemed, were to leave for Saigon the following morning.

That morning Elizabeth and I decided to go out together to do some shopping as we knew that we would not be seeing any decent shops again for a long time. We took a rickshaw to the Army and Navy Stores and then coming back along Chowringhee decided to turn off into a marketplace which we had noticed previously. It was much cooler strolling through the shaded market and we were immediately adopted by a small grinning boy carrying a basket almost as big as himself. We told him he was wasting his time, that we could easily carry all that we were likely to buy, but he still grinned and hung on. He accompanied us into all the shops we entered while we looked at various merchandise, discussed prices and bought nothing.

"Look, Junior," I said patiently. "Run along, that's a good *chicco*. We are only looking. We have no money. You'll just be losing business if you hang around us," but that did not deter him. He grinned and continued to cling like a limpet. A couple of American corporals also did the same, but we did not notice that at first. We only noticed it when they asked our advice about the price and quality of silk stockings. They asked if we thought the stockings were worth what was being asked. We looked at the stockings and said it was far too much.

"Good full-fashioned stockings, very expensive," the merchant whined.

"I know that," I replied, "But those stockings are no more fully fashioned than you are, you old rogue."

"Well, thanks for putting us straight about that," the taller of the two corporals said. "Say, would you mind if we kinda trailed along with you, ma'am? You see we just got back from Burma and we're on our way back to the States. Maybe you would help us pick out decent gifts to take back home. It's easy for guys like us to be taken in."

Put like that, of course, we could not refuse. They may have been shooting a line, but it always broke our hearts to see the troops buying a lot of junk at exorbitant prices. We could imagine their womenfolk at home trying to enthuse over cheap, orange stockings and blouses that would not stand one washing, badly-cut underwear and old-fashioned handbags. We advised them about several purchases and they bought some very nice lengths of silk, four handbags, six embroidered blouses, and several brass and ivory souvenirs.

They embarrassed us by wanting to buy things for us, but we refused to allow them. The tall one, who was called Hank, was the more talkative of the two. He said it was two years since he had bought a gift for a pretty girl and he had lots of money, so I suggested that he spend it on the folks at home.

"Gee, what would you do with such dames," he asked the grinning boy with the basket, who was still hanging around and gradually getting his basket filled up. Soon Junior's basket was completely full and he was urging the Americans to buy flowers for us at a tiny flower shop.

"Say that's an idea," Hank agreed and turning to me, said, "Say, you can't refuse to let us buy corsages for the two of you, can you? I mean, just because you've been so swell about all this stuff, and because you've got such lovely blue eyes."

"But we can't wear flowers with uniform," I protested.

"Sure you can. It'll pep it up," he said, unabashed. "Besides I haven't seen a girl with blue eyes for two years."

Laughing, we all went into the shop and Hank selected the flowers he wanted and the proprietor made up two small identical corsages. After they had been pinned on us, Hank asked Junior if he liked them. Junior nodded so Hank paid for them. Elizabeth and the other boy walked ahead, so we followed them, and Junior followed us. Suddenly Hank stopped and wrinkling his nose said, "I don't like it."

"Don't like what?" I asked.

"The corsage," he replied.

"But it's very pretty," I protested.

But he was unconvinced and turning to Junior said, "Listen, don't you think it's a crime to buy white flowers for a girl with such lovely blue eyes?"

Junior had no idea what he was talking about so he nodded and grinned.

"I knew you'd agree," Hank said, pleased. "C'mon—we're going back."

In spite of my protestations we went back to the shop and Hank requested the florist to make up a corsage to match my eyes. Feeling extremely foolish, I sat on a rickety stool which was placed at my disposal while the florist picked out flowers which would match my eyes.

With transaction completed and Junior's approval sought, we again left the shop and set off to find the other two, but again Hank stopped, looked at the corsage and declared he didn't like it.

"Oh! What's the matter now?" I asked.

He turned to Junior. "We made a mistake, kid," he said. "Just take a look. See what I mean? It just isn't possible to match eyes like that and we had no right to try." By this time Elizabeth and the other corporal had come back to find out what had happened to us. They found me seated in the flower shop, surrounded by Hank, the florist, and Junior. Eventually I came out wearing a corsage of tiny pink rosebuds and said that I was not going to be bullied into any further changes.

We walked a few steps and Hank paused and looked at me quizzically. "I like that," he said.

"Well thank goodness for that," I laughed.

They walked back to the hotel with us and left us there. The last we saw of them, they were striding swiftly through the crowded arcade with Junior's skinny brown legs trotting after them, his loaded basket on his head.

Mildred went swimming after lunch, but Elizabeth and I decided to pack our bags and take a nap. The R.T.O. had arranged transport to the station for us at twenty after four, but at four o'clock Mildred had not returned and her belongings were strewn all over the room, giving it the appearance of a bargain basement after a January sale. At ten minutes past four she came back and asked for the iron as she had some things to press. I told her the iron was at the bottom of my trunk and she had better get busy with her packing.

That was Mildred all over. She seemed to have no conception of time. Somehow or other we managed to gather up her scattered possessions and cram them into her various bags and trunks. What would not go in we rolled into her bedding roll and at 4:27 we were actually in the truck surrounded by all our belongings. The R.T.O. was fluttering around like a Victorian nanny and the truck was about to depart when Fay suddenly noticed that Mildred was no longer with us. That also was typical of Mildred. No one ever saw her go but she was never where she should have been at a given time. The R.T.O. was a busy man, the heat was overpowering, he was tired of India and he was really exasperated.

"Then you will have to go without her," he snapped.

"But she has our travel warrants," we said. "She's in charge of us."

I thought the R.T.O. was about to have an apoplectic fit, but he took a firm grip on himself and sent people off in all directions to look for her. Jill was positive she knew where Mildred would be so she climbed out of the truck and ran back into the hotel.

Finally Mildred was found in a telephone booth in the lobby of the hotel and dragged, protesting, from it. The R.T.O. lifted her into the truck and we were about to set off when we realized that Jill had not returned, so forbidding anyone to move, the R.T.O. went to look for her himself.

"She wasn't where I thought she would be," Jill was saying as he brought her back. Looking at the R.T.O. at that moment I felt sure that if he was not already a married man, he never would be. Eventually we were on our way to Howrah Station, all of us telling Mildred off in no uncertain manner, but she was quite unruffled. "There's lots of time," she said. "And anyway, I promised to call Ken before I left. He's such a sweet kid."

Accommodation on the train was very limited, and the five of us were crammed into a two-berth compartment with all of our luggage packed in around us. Another two-berth compartment was being vacated a few stations ahead and two of us could then move in there. Goodness knows how many people were on the platform to see us off and there were only a few minutes to spare when we again realized that Mildred was missing.

"If she didn't have our tickets I wouldn't care where she got to," Fay said at the end of her patience. "In fact I would urge her to lose herself."

Elizabeth, although herself exasperated by Mildred's scattiness, felt called upon to defend her fellow-Canadian and it looked as though there might be a first-class row between Elizabeth and Fay. Actually the train had started to pull out of the platform when Mildred was passed feet first through the window by Keith and an unidentified man.

We all turned on her then. "Don't get excited, kids,' she said calmly. "I'm here, aren't I? You see, I saw a couple of sergeants whom I met at the swimming pool this afternoon, so I had to go and say good-bye to them. They were such sweet kids."

"Keep calm, everyone," I said. "Keep calm. As she says, she's here and it's too hot to argue. But don't do it again," I added menacingly, fixing Mildred with a glare.

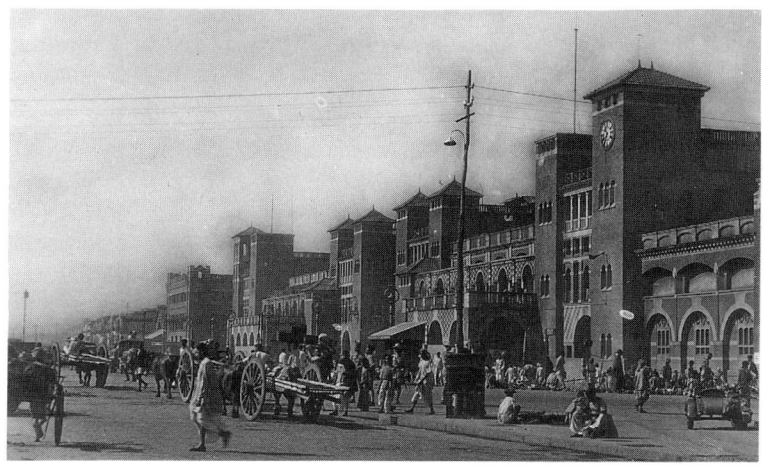

Howrah Station, Calcutta

The journey was uneventful. We left the train for dinner about half past nine that night, leaving a coolie in charge of our compartment and at dinner met an army matron who was traveling on the same train. She asked if one of us would be kind enough to share her compartment for the night as she was rather nervous about traveling alone, so we saw to it that Mildred volunteered to do so. Surely, even she could not possibly go astray under the eagle eye of an army matron and we considered it a fitting punishment for the run-around she had given us. After dinner, Elizabeth and I had our luggage moved into the compartment which had been vacated further down the train and then we settled down for the night.

We changed trains at Muri the following morning and arrived in Ranchi during the afternoon. We checked in at the R.T.O.'s office on Ranchi station and asked him to arrange transport for us to our respective hospitals. He consulted a list and said we were all five going to the Combined Military Hospital (C.M.H.) there since the 75 General Hospital was on the move. He thought the whole hospital was going to Malaya, so it looked as though Elizabeth, Mildred and I would be on the move again very shortly.

Chapter Eight

The matron of the Combined Military Hospital was pleased to see Jill and Fay, but she was anything but pleased to see the three of us. In fact, she told us pointblank that she objected to her hospital being used as a transit camp for the 75 General Hospital. We disliked her intensely and soon found that the feeling was general throughout the hospital. She said there was really no room for us and we would have to share bungalows with her permanent staff and it would be very inconvenient.

From the matron's office we went to the quarters and introduced ourselves to a very harassed nurse who was in charge of the mess. She put me in a bungalow immediately opposite the matron's with a girl named Mary Purvis. Fortunately, she did not seem to consider me the nuisance that the matron did and gave me a very warm welcome. She helped me unpack and made space for me in the wardrobe and drawers. We shared that bungalow for several weeks and we were like old friends from the beginning. Her husband, a friendly young captain, came in during the afternoon, and after being introduced to him, he invited me to a party in his mess the following evening. It was about seventy miles away through the jungle but he was sure it would be enjoyable and transport could be arranged both ways.

The bungalow was not too bad and certainly a vast improvement on those we had in Kalyan. There were two big rooms, one of which we used as a bathroom. Water was rationed since it had to be brought in from quite a distance each day. Often we had to wash in the same water more than once, but enough warm water was carried in for us each evening for a bath. The bearer filled our thermos flasks with drinking water each morning.

The morning after arriving in Ranchi we went on duty. I was assigned to the operating theater and was not off duty in time to go to Captain Purvis's party, but Elizabeth and Mildred went. During the afternoon the matron from 75 General Hospital came to see us. She was leaving for Malaya within the next few hours. Mildred, Elizabeth, and I were all introduced to her at the same time. She took all our particulars and then shook hands warmly saying that she would be looking forward to seeing us again in Malaya. "You will find we are a very happy family at the seventy-five," she said. We liked her and walked back to our wards with light hearts. We felt sure that moving to Malaya with the seventy-five would be wonderful, but that was as far as it got.

Three weeks after arriving in Ranchi, the matron of C.M.H., much to everyone's delight, went home for demobilization. She smiled at me for the first time when she shook hands outside my bungalow and said she hoped I would be happy in Malaya. I asked her if anything definite had come through yet but she said no it had not.

Miss Astridge, the assistant matron, whom everyone liked, was then in temporary charge and we persuaded her to try and find out what was happening regarding our transfer. All our letters were going to the seventy-five and taking ages to catch up with us. At the time of course we did not know that and could not understand why we were not getting any letters. Headquarters, in New Delhi, thinking we were already with the seventy-five, kept on sending our letters there. Major Stanton, the registrar at the hospital, also did what he could for us in his slow and rather silly way. He also issued us with various documents which we would need on the journey, and did not seem to mind one bit when he got my thumb prints on Mildred's documents and hers on mine.

However, three months after arriving in Ranchi, we were still on the temporary staff of the C.M.H. but Fay and Jill, who had been placed on the permanent staff there, were in Malaya, which proves that the British Army will always muddle through somehow.

Taken on the whole, we were quite happy in Ranchi. We had a good club there and a nice crowd of people. There were a couple of weddings in the mess and we went to Government House several times. Elizabeth had an affair with a Royal Air Force fellow and assured us that it was the "real thing" this time. It always was. Mildred unearthed Larry Tennant, a character whom she had met on the ship coming out to India, in the Rup-a-Sree Cinema one night and arranged to go and meet him at a dance in the Young Women's Christian Association (YWCA).

The YWCA in Ranchi was a delightful place where we could get wonderful meals at reasonable prices and where we spent many happy hours. Meeting Larry there was like meeting a friend from home and we often saw him after that. I felt sorry for him as he was still carrying the torch for a nurse with whom he had fallen in love on board ship, but she had since married a tea planter.

It was at the YWCA that Larry introduced us to a friend of his, whose name, other than "Tiny" I cannot remember. He was a big, coarse fellow with a heart of gold, but, unfortunately, a love for the bottle. For some reason or other, Mildred seemed to think that Tiny was a "sweet kid" and took him under her wing.

Larry was in charge of the army mobile cinema unit in Ranchi and ran off films for us at the rest center whenever we asked him. He also had a jeep at his disposal which proved to be very useful on numerous occasions.

In October a new matron arrived and she would not allow the staff to go out after duty on any night when they were on duty until nine o'clock. This meant that I had to sneak out the back way if I wanted to go anywhere after late duty. The girls always sympathized with me because my bungalow was immediately opposite the matron's. One night there was a dance which I particularly wanted to attend. Mildred was going with Tiny and, since she had come off duty at five o'clock that day, went openly with him in a rickshaw, but I had to sneak out in the pitch dark to where Larry had parked his jeep, so that the matron could neither see nor hear it.

Jim Berry, my escort, met me at the back door of the bungalow, Mary having bolted it behind me, and led me through the trees to the jeep. It was necessary to back the jeep a little before I could get into it and suddenly I stepped back into space and found myself lying at the bottom of a monsoon trench.

"Where's Eve?" I heard Larry ask.

"I don't know." Jim sounded very alarmed. "She was here a second ago and then she seemed to vanish into thin air."

"Here I am," I called faintly as soon as I could get my breath.

Jim jumped in beside me and lifted me up to Larry, then climbed out himself. They set me right way up, brushed me down and put me in the jeep, but it quite spoiled my evening.

Jim Berry was a physiotherapist in charge of the rehabilitation department at a neighboring hospital. He had a wonderfully equipped department there and many repatriated prisoners of war passed through his capable hands. The hospital was in a beautiful setting and even boasted a swimming pool where I spent so many happy hours as Jim's guest. Jim's manner was charming and natural. War-shattered prisoners seemed to have confidence in him almost at once. Many of them, in a remarkably short space of time, were mastering new artificial limbs and returning to England. Several who had spent long, unhappy years in prison camps were terrified of meeting strangers and it was wonderful to see how Jim helped them to overcome even that.

Off duty he was the same natural, pleasant-mannered individual and danced with the easy grace of the trained athlete that he was. Without exceptions he was the best dancing partner I ever had in India.

Jim had been in India for three and a half years, so I was not surprised when he told me in October that he was going home. Naturally I was pleased for his sake but he said he did not want to go.

"Why ever not?" I gasped.

He said that he had always been happy in India and that he loved the job he was doing. His mother had died when he was very young and his father had been killed in a raid over Birmingham. He had no brothers or sisters, in fact, no one. "Besides which," he added, "I happen to be in love with you."

As I looked at him I wondered why I was not in love with him as he had all the qualities that the average woman looks for in a man. I thought of Louise, strangely, and wondered if I was being "standoffish" again.

"Jim, you may feel very differently about all this when you get back to England," I pointed out to him. "You have met so few English girls out here, you know, and you may have forgotten how nice and plentiful they are."

I promised to write to him and to see him and talk things over when we were both back in England and able to think more rationally.

He was still in Ranchi, however, when the C.M.H. had to vacate the premises in November. We moved forty miles to Ramgarh. Elizabeth, Mildred, and I, still being on the temporary staff, moved with the hospital. It was a very hectic week before we left, packing up on the wards and transferring patients to neighboring hospitals. Off duty, we packed our own possessions and said our good-byes.

I was in the last transport that drove through the gates and from the back of the truck looked back on the deserted bungalows with a pang of regret. A group of unhappy looking rickshaw boys stood at the gates as we passed. I waved and they waved back.

"Poor devils, they'll miss you," Major Stanton, who was seated beside me, said.

"Yes. Trade won't be so brisk for them without us," I agreed.

The forty mile journey by road was very pleasant and we passed hardly any habitations at all. We arrived in Ramgarh in the heat of midday and although much higher, it was much hotter than it had been in Ranchi. The hospital buildings were long wooden huts and looked very crude after the imposing buildings we had occupied at St. Paul's School in Ranchi. They were spread over a very large area. The sisters' mess could be reached either by going much further along the main road or by taking a short cut between the hospital buildings. Later, when the wards were occupied, we were not allowed to drive any vehicle between the hospital buildings after eight o'clock at night.

Everywhere there was chaos. The advance party had nothing ready for us and the servants who had been brought from Ranchi walked out en masse, refusing to live in such an out-of-the-way place. There was furniture in the dining room and in the lounge but none in the bungalows, which were set in straight parallel rows, eight to a row, with long verandahs back and front from end to end.

We found that we would have no need to double up here as there were enough bungalows for us to have one each, so we sorted ourselves out. Once again we were without a matron, the new one having been posted to Singapore only a few days before, so again Astridge was in command. A new sister who had recently arrived from England was in charge of the mess. She had come with the advance party and was by then almost on the verge of a nervous breakdown, having had

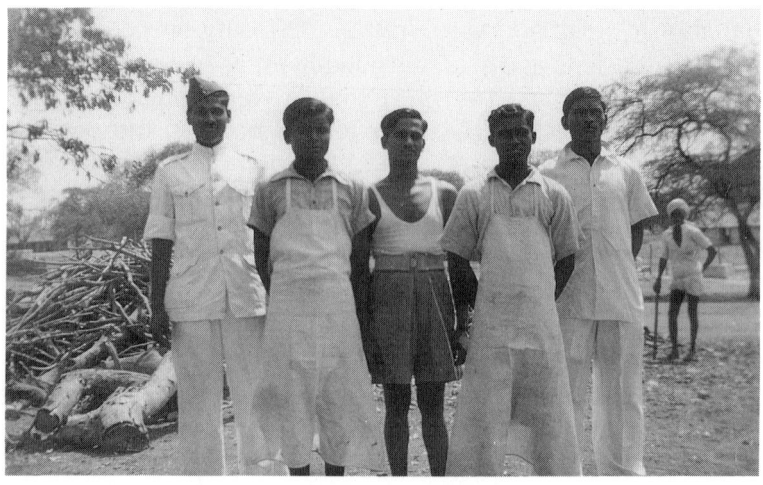

Mess Servants

such a trying time both with the servants and the highly temperamental quartermaster. We all felt sorry for her and helped her as much as we could. Since we were not getting any patients for a few days we were free to get both the quarters and the wards ready without hindrance.

There was an empty bungalow next to mine which was to be occupied by the new matron when she arrived, so once again I was to be alarmingly close to authority. On the other side of me was Betty Tappin, a sweet shy girl, with whom I had been quite friendly in Ranchi. All the bungalows had electric ceiling fans and built-in wardrobes. There was also a tiny wash place with a zinc bath in each bungalow. Alternate bungalows had the unheard-of luxury of a cold water tap—but mostly lukewarm—and the greatest luxury of all was a row of sewered toilets quite a distance from the quarters but well worth the walk there.

By bedtime, Betty and I had the most orderly bungalows in the place. We had obtained curtains for the doors and windows from the Red Cross store, where Miss Astridge had put us to work during the afternoon. Between us, we had stealthily removed from debris scattered all over the place, two bedside tables and a big chipped table. Our trunks were used as dressing tables and our clothes had been put away in the wardrobes. Another visit to the Red Cross store when no one was around unearthed a few covers for the tables and trunks. We had no beds so we spread our bedding rolls on the floor and slept like babies all night.

The next day, furniture, beds and mattresses arrived and the place began to look more habitable. We managed to recruit a few servants from the village but could not get any fresh meat or much variety in food. For two weeks our diet seemed to consist mainly of corned beef, canned turnips and jellies, but at least it was always beautifully served. To make matters worse, there were no restaurants where we could go for a decent meal and there was no entertainment.

In some ways it was worse than Kalyan, but once we got organized there were frequent trips to Ranchi on any vehicle going there and numerous messes in the area arranged transport to many activities. We often traveled seventy miles merely to go out to dinner.

Soon the patients began to arrive and we were back to normal ward routine. With the American army having been in occupation there previously, we had the most modern operating theater we had seen since we left England and every ward had an electric refrigerator.

Soon after we arrived in Ramgarh, Betty, Elizabeth and I went on night duty under the command of one of the most unpleasant sisters imaginable. We called her "Dizzy Dora" among ourselves. Poor Dizzy Dora was a born muddler. She could never remember where she put things, had no idea of organization, whined, nagged and panicked continuously. She was madly in love with one of the doctors who avoided her like the plague. Fortunately for me, Dora had a morbid dread of dysentery and I saw very little of her as one of my wards was the dysentery ward.

Life in Ramgarh was decidedly dull on nightduty. In other places there had been an officers' club with a swimming pool and other amenities within easy reach and there we had relaxed between coming off duty in the mornings and going to bed. Now it was just bed and work with a constitutional walk to the village every morning.

In the village we were struck by the shining cleanliness of the few shops and made friends with all the shopkeepers. Business was never brisk in such a remote village and often there was a lengthy interval between entering a shop and asking to see certain wares. The interval was occupied by dusting chairs for us, placing cigarettes and matches at our disposal, and asking solicitously about our health, our bowels and our relatives.

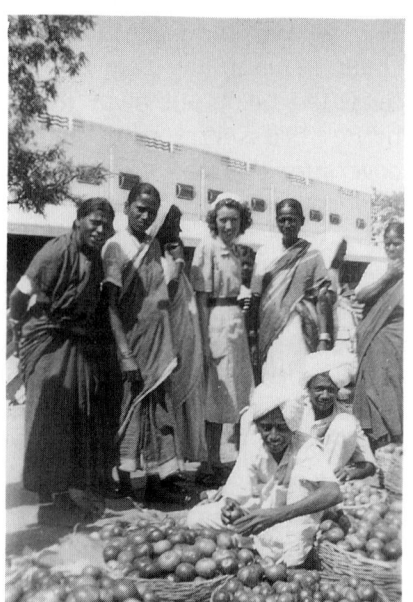

Buying fruit from the locals

Each morning we visited the only fruit shop in the village where, even if we only bought the smallest quantity of fruit possible between the three of us, the dear white-bearded proprietor pinned a tiny wet rose on each of our dresses.

During our spell of night duty, we hardly saw an English face apart from the hospital staff. We never had time off during night duty, which lasted a month. Although it was so terribly hot during the days, the nights in Ramgarh were bitterly cold now that it was winter. As I huddled inside my cape trying to keep warm during the long watches of the night, I comforted myself with the thought of the long leave I was going to take in Mussorrie over the Christmas and New Year's period with Bill. He was still in Delhi and kept reminding me in letters that I had promised to go there with him when I was entitled to a long leave. I was actually long past being entitled to a long leave but the opportunity of getting away for one had never arisen. My leave with Bill also was not to be. Two weeks after going on night duty a letter from him informed me that he had suddenly been posted to Singapore and he asked if I would try to get a posting there too.

It must have been about five o'clock one morning when I heard a jeep drive noisily through the hospital grounds and come to a halt outside the duty room window of my ward. Wondering who could be stupid enough to drive through the grounds at that hour, I decided to investigate when I heard Mildred's pronounced Canadian accent say, "Well, gee, thanks a lot. It sure was nice of you to bring me back and I do appreciate it." Then I heard the indistinct tones of a man in reply. I wondered who on earth Mildred could be with and what sort of scrape she had got into this time.

When I got outside to the jeep Mildred had gone and a military provost captain was just getting back into the jeep. I pointed out to him that it was against hospital orders to drive through the grounds between the hours of 8 P.M. and 8 A.M.

"There are patients sleeping in all these wards," I said.

"I'm very sorry," he said. "But surely Miss James should have told me, shouldn't she?"

"She certainly should," I replied. I sensed that he was in a bad temper about something and I asked socially if he had far to go and if he would like a cup of tea. He said that was an excellent idea; he would love a cup of tea as he was very cold and not looking forward to the drive back to Ranchi. I led him into the duty room and asked him to be seated, then I went to ask my ward boy to make some tea. I thought then it might be a good idea to go and find Dizzy Dora in case she walked in on our little tête-à-tête and misconstrued it. I explained to the captain that I was going to see the night sister. "But please don't tell her who your friend is."

"Friend?" he burst out. "She's no friend of mine. One of my men came to me in the middle of the night and said he had found her wandering around in Ranchi. What else could I do but get out of bed and drive her to her hospital myself?" I realized now why he was in a bad temper and was more curious than ever to find out what Mildred had been up to. "Anyway," he added, "I certainly wouldn't want to get the girl into any sort of row, so I won't give her away."

Dora was taking a nap in one of the empty side wards on Betty's ward, a habit of hers, so I went in and told her briefly what had happened. "It's all right for me to give him some tea isn't it, sister?" I asked.

"Oh yes, of course," she replied. "But who did you say it was he brought?"

"I didn't say," I said sweetly. "You see, she had already gone to the quarters by the time I got outside to find out who was driving through the grounds at that hour." I had still not given Mildred away, nor had I told a lie.

Dora, I knew, was simply bursting with curiosity and got off the bed and started pulling on her shoes. "I'll come and join you. I'm dying for a cup of tea," she said. Dizzy Dora never missed any opportunity to meet a man or to get any gossip. I introduced her to the provost captain. She was all charm and gush, but almost immediately she asked who the girl was whom he had driven home.

Behind Dora's back I put my finger to my lips, so with a perfectly straight face he said, "I really don't know, sister. One of my men found her somehow or other in Ranchi about two o'clock this morning and I couldn't do anything else but bring her here myself. Believe me, under the circumstances, I was not interested in such social pleasantries as finding out her name. All I was interested in was getting her here as soon as possible and getting back to my place to catch up on some sleep."

"No, I suppose not," Dora agreed. "But I wish you had asked her name because we really should take disciplinary action, you know. These girls have to be kept under control."

"Yes, I quite see that," he agreed. "And I'm sorry now that I didn't find out for you."

"Was she a Q.A. or a V.A.D.?" Dora persisted.

"I really don't know," he said. "She was wearing civilian clothing."

"Was there anything about her you would recognize again," Dora quizzed on. "I mean her height or figure or whether she spoke in any particular dialect."

"No, I'm afraid not," the captain lied. "I say, sister, this tea is delicious. It just hits the right spot."

As he shook hands with me on departing he winked broadly and I thanked him with a smile. Although annoyed, he had been a good sport about the whole thing.

I managed to find time to run down to Mildred's bungalow before she went to breakfast.

"Whatever did you get up to last night," I wanted to know.

She went into a long tale of woe which was very complicated. She had got a lift into Ranchi the previous evening to meet Tiny and they had a "swell time" until he became the worse for wear after too many drinks. Finally he had passed out cold and when she went to find a telephone or a taxi, leaving him sleeping comfortably in the street, he had been found by a couple of military policemen and carted off by them. Mildred, finding him no longer where she had left him, was sure he must have been kidnapped and panicked. It was by this time after one o'clock in the morning.

"I wandered around scared stiff and not seeing a living soul until I stopped an army jeep and then I was taken to military police headquarters or somewhere," she said. It all sounded very disjointed and mixed up and I had to get back to my duties before Dizzy Dora started checking up on me.

"Anyway, I covered up for you," I said. "Dora is dying to know who it was so that she can make trouble but the captain pretended that he didn't know your name and had no idea what you looked like or anything, so remember that and for heaven's sake don't give yourself away."

"Gee, I wouldn't think of it," Mildred assured me. "Thanks a lot for being so swell about it. I'm sure through with that Tiny now."

Mildred went on duty at eight o'clock that morning. She worked on the same ward that Elizabeth was on at night. She burst into the duty room where Elizabeth sat writing the night report, and said quickly, "Gee, you know I went to Ranchi last night and I didn't get back till five o'clock this morning. Boy, am I tired!"

Elizabeth, who had already been briefed by me, tried to signal and to stop her flow of conversation, but it was Mildred's own fault. She should have seen Dora standing at the medicine cupboard.

Food continued to be very poor in the mess and if we, on night duty, had not sustained ourselves at our own expense, we would never have been able to sleep during the day. After our walk to the village in the mornings we used to sit on the verandah and consume vast quantities of cornflakes, canned cream, and fruit. Then during the night I was fed very generously by my ward boy.

That came about because of an insane patient who was under my care. He was in a private ward immediately opposite the duty room where I spent most of the night. Being insane and a criminal he had an armed guard. Neither the guard nor the patient could speak a word of English, nor could they speak Urdu to any great extent, at least not my brand of Urdu, so communication between us was impossible. The guard had a disconcerting habit of falling asleep with his rifle between his legs and, as the patient slept hardly ever, I had many nasty moments which were quite a strain on my nerves.

I was glad to have the talkative ward boy in for a chat. He usually dropped in soon after Dizzy Dora's midnight round. At least he did most of the chatting; I just listened. Indian fashion, he told me the most embarrassing details about his own and his relatives' lives. Often I thought I would scream if I had to hear any more about his father's wretched bowels, his son's prominent navel, or his wife's tendency towards nymphomania. Actually, I know I should not have encouraged him, but when one has an insane patient and a sleeping guard with a loaded rifle within five yards, any kind of human contact is welcome, even Mukan Lal.

One night in an unguarded moment I happened to mention to Mukan Lal that I liked Indian food, and as a result he brought me his ration of curry and rice every night. Goodness knows how or under what conditions it was cooked; I just didn't dare think about that. And I couldn't throw it away because he always stood over me in delighted admiration until I had eaten every scrap.

In return I offered whatever food I had brought from the mess in my tiffin carrier but he, rather tactlessly I thought, told me what he thought of English food.

Mukan Lal of course wanted to know all about me. Was I married? Why not? I must be very old. Twenty-one? Pooh! An Indian girl at my age would have four, five, six babies. Why did not someone marry me? By English standards, he admitted grudgingly, that I was not bad-looking, certainly good enough for English officer sahibs. I may have been overly-sensitive, but he seemed to infer that English office sahibs were not too fussy.

Dizzy Dora seemed to dislike poor Mukan Lal from the very first and never gave him a moment's peace. Goodness knows why, and I began to think that one night she would be attacked by him in the dark, she goaded him so much. But fortunately for all of us, she fell over an open drain one morning and twisted her ankle. That was the end of her night duty with us and Sister Tunney came on in her place. After that we had a very busy spell. I had to take over surgery as well as dysentery and convalescent, because there were some very bad petrol burn cases which needed constant attention. So much extra work under Dora's supervision would have been too much for me, but with the fat comfortable Tunney in charge, things went along smoothly and happily.

There were lots of jackals in the jungle around the hospital and we used to hear them howling all night long. Frequently we saw them roaming around the grounds scavenging for food and one of them attacked Tunney one night. Fortunately, it was only about nine o'clock and it was immediately outside the British Other Ranks' ward. Some of the boys who were convalescent dashed out when they heard her scream and threw stones at it. The guard appeared and shot at it. We thought he wounded it but were not really sure. Tunney was shaken but that was all.

Elizabeth's R.A.F. friend flew back to England while we were on night duty. My leave with Bill was out of the question, so Elizabeth and I decided to take a few days off if we could tack them onto the days off we were entitled to after night duty, and spend Christmas in Calcutta. Then, about February, we might be able to manage a longer leave in Darjeeling or Kashmir. Betty said she would like to join us too, so we set about making plans. Since this was to be the first peacetime Christmas since the end of the war, we decided to make it as much like a prewar Christmas at home as we could. We even decided that we would hang up our stockings which the other two could fill, but, as usual, our plans went awry.

On December 12 we read in hospital orders that Mildred, Elizabeth, and I were transferred to the permanent staff of the Combined Military Hospital, Ramgarh, effective from December 11. On December 13 we were all posted separately, I to Secunderabad, Elizabeth to Chhindwara, Mildred and another girl called Joan Goodwin to Dehra Dun, and Betty to Assam. We were all to leave Ramgarh within a week.

It was a shock to be parted just at Christmastime after being together for so long, but there was nothing we could do about it. Our new matron had arrived and was unsympathetic. Mary Purvis wanted to go to Secunderabad in my place as her husband, by this time, was somewhere near there, but they would not listen to her. Anyway when the time came she was too ill to make the journey. She tried to pass it off but the morning I left Ramgarh she became a patient in the hospital. It was her fifth attack of amoebic dysentery, and that meant repatriation to England.

Mildred and Joan Goodwin were the first to leave. We went to the station at Bakakhana to see them off on the train to Calcutta, where they would change for Delhi and so on up north to Dehra Dun, from there it was said, they would be able to see snowcapped mountains. How we envied them.

Elizabeth was the next to leave but Betty was detained for a further week since the registrar had not been able to make reservations for her all the way to Assam, so she was still on night duty. However, when Elizabeth left, Betty insisted on getting up early so that we could all go to the station and wave Elizabeth off to Chhindwara. Poor Betty looked so dejected that we all wept.

Chapter Nine

The following day I left for Secunderabad. It was the first time I had ever undertaken a long train journey in India alone and I was very apprehensive about it since riots had broken out in recent weeks. The fact that a British nurse had only a few days before been found murdered in a first-class compartment on the Bengal-Nagpur Railway did nothing to alleviate my fears. What was even worse to me was the realization that for the first peacetime Christmas I was to be separated from the colleagues to whom I had become so attached during the time we had been in India.

One becomes resigned to these things in service life though. Making a pretense of eating lunch was difficult and as soon as I could, I made my escape from the dining room to go back to my bungalow. Betty came in soon afterward looking thoroughly miserable.

"All ready?" she asked in a hollow voice.

"Yes, all ready," I replied. "I wish the ambulance or whatever is taking us to the station would come. I'm fed up of prolonging the agony. I gave you my home address, didn't I?"

"Yes, don't worry, Eve. If those damned Indians murder you on the way I'll get your folks to kick up such a stink in Whitehall. They should never send us on these long journeys without escorts while all these riots are going on. Even the men aren't safe. John said he and a couple of other fellows had to threaten to shoot at a crowd of congress *wallahs* in Muzzafurpur station last week. It's time all the British were recalled from India. The war's over now and it would do them good to stew in their own juices. Give the silly fatheads a chance to see if they can govern themselves." Calm, quiet Betty was letting herself get worked up about the whole thing.

"What annoys me," I said, "is the stupidity of not allowing us outside the compound after dark without a British escort and then pushing us off on these journeys from one end of India to the other all alone."

"Oh, that's the army all over," Betty said in disgust.

"Wonder if the rioters will cut my throat or just beat me to death," I said musingly.

"Eve, don't," Betty said with a long shudder.

"Seester Porter," a soft voice called from the doorway and I turned to see the fat, bearded Sikh *havildar* from the Registrar's office. He was holding out my travel warrant.

"Major Stanton sahib send," he said.

"Thanks, *havildar*," I said taking it. "Did he say anything about an escort for me?"

"No, seester sahib," he said, with a great display of perfect teeth. "Escort is not necessary."

"That's what you think," I said between my teeth.

"It is quite simple journey," he said patiently. "Why one of my *chiccos* could find his way there."

"Then by all means send one in my place," I said brutally.

He laughed indulgently as if to say these English half-wits must have their little joke.

"Major Stanton sahib, he fix everything good," he went on. "First you take train at Bakakhana at a quarter after two, then you get out at ten o'clock tonight in Tatanagur and go straight to R.T.O."

"Who?"

"The railway traffic officer."

"Oh, and what will he do?" I asked. "Put the flags out?"

Again the indulgent little laugh. "No, he put you on midnight train for Bombay," he said.

I brightened up at that. "Oh, I go to Bombay, do I?"

"No, seester. You stay on Bombay train until you get to Kazipet on Tuesday afternoon, then from there you go to R.T.O."

"He will keep cropping up won't he?" Betty chipped in.

"Not same R.T.O.," the *havildar* said. "The R.T.O. at Kazipet—if there is one."

"What do you mean, 'if there is one?'" I exploded.

"Kazipet very small station," he replied. "So perhaps no R.T.O. and if no R.T.O. you go to station master and he fix you up."

"Fix me up with what?" I asked suspiciously.

"With train for Secunderabad," the *havildar* said bringing out his words much as a conjurer brings a rabbit out of a hat.

"Oh, so it's as simple as that is it?" I said. "All I do is change at Tatanagur tonight and at Kazipet on Tuesday afternoon."

"That is all," the *havildar* said, obviously relieved that he had at last driven his point home. "Major Stanton sahib he fix everything. He send telegrams to both stations telling them to watch out for you and to reserve compartments on trains."

I thanked the *havildar* and dismissed him. "It doesn't sound too difficult, does it?" I asked, turning to Betty.

"Everything sounds fine except for the fact that Major Stanton has fixed it," Betty said bitterly. "It's a good thing Mary Bowden is going on the same train to Calcutta."

I was glad about that, too. If there was time she would see me onto the train at Tatanagur and her Urdu was far better than mine.

At that moment I heard Mary calling along the verandah that our conveyance was ready. Betty burst into tears and flung her arms about my neck as a couple of servants came in to carry my baggage out to the truck. It was a dilapidated fifteen hundredweight truck and Mary was making quite a fuss about it.

"Why didn't they send the *pani* (water) wagon for us?" She was demanding angrily, "then we could have dressed up for the occasion in a couple of dirty saris."

When the baggage had been stacked on the truck we managed to squash in beside the Indian army driver. Then just as we were leaving, Jane Dunn, one of the sisters, dashed up to say that her fiancé was traveling on the same train to Calcutta and to look out for him at the station. We promised we would as Donald, being an official on the railway, would no doubt be a great asset to us.

So, in a cloud of dust, we set off along the bumpy, sandy road to Bakakhana, and for whatever lay ahead.

The train was already in the station when we got there and, true enough, a first-class compartment had been reserved for us. So far Major Stanton was in favor. We found Donald in the company of a Royal Air Force officer in the next compartment. Tea was served at Muri, a small station in Bihar province, and dinner was served when we got to Tatanagur just after ten o'clock.

Leaving a coolie in charge of our baggage the four of us went together to the station restaurant. I was the only one leaving the train here and felt rather sorry as I would have liked to be going on to Calcutta again. With dinner over, Donald set off to find the R.T.O. for me and to arrange my transfer to the Bombay mail train. The train for Calcutta was not due to leave for about fifteen minutes.

A few moments later Donald returned, looking very harassed and accompanied by a tall British sergeant with R.T.O. on his sleeve.

"This the lady?" the sergeant asked, looking at Mary.

"No, I am," I said. "I understand that accommodation has been booked for me on the midnight train for Bombay. Major Stanton of the C.M.H. Ramgarh contacted you about it."

The sergeant looked puzzled. "I've never heard of Major Stanton," he said, "and I didn't even know there was a military hospital in Ramgarh. Anyway, you couldn't travel on that train because it's for civilians only."

Our dear major sank even lower in my estimation, if that were possible. "Major Stanton, should, in my opinion, be sent home quickly," I said bitterly. "He's been exposed to the Indian sun far too long. Sergeant, isn't there anything you can do about getting me on that train?"

"Wait here a minute and I'll go and see what the station master can do," the sergeant said. "Would you like to come along sir?" he asked Donald.

When they returned it seemed that between them they had somehow arranged for me to be accommodated on the train. That was something of a relief; so I saw Mary, Donald, and Bill back to their train, fished out my possessions and stood and waved them off.

It was very lonely after they had gone, but fighting down my fears, I got a couple of coolies to take my baggage to the waiting room. It was bitterly cold and the waiting room was small, smelly, and uninspiring. It never failed to astonish me to find how cold it could become in India at nighttime after the stifling heat of the day.

True to his word, the sergeant put me on the Bombay train as soon as it came in. I was in a compartment in which there were four berths, two of them already occupied.

"You should be all right now, sister," the sergeant said after my baggage had been put aboard and he had spread out my bedding roll for me on one of the upper berths. "You'll be safe in Bombay on Wednesday morning."

"But I'm not going to Bombay," I said as the train began to move.

"Where are you going?" he asked looking concerned, and running along beside the moving train.

"I'm going to Secunderabad," I shouted through the open window, "and I have to change at Kazipet."

"But this train doesn't go to Kazipet," he yelled as the train gathered speed. "You'll have to change at Manmod."

The sergeant's worried face gradually disappeared from sight and I was left alone with my thoughts. One of my sleeping companions was snoring loudly, but the other, a pretty little Anglo-Indian girl, who was on the berth below mine, smiled sweetly and introduced herself. Her name was Margaret.

Scrambling up to my berth, I must have fallen asleep almost at once to dream that Major Stanton was sick and I was giving him an intramuscular injection with a blunt needle. It must have been about seven o'clock the next morning when I woke up to find that unfortunately, it was only a dream after all.

Margaret was dressed and moving around quietly gathering her possessions together. I noticed that she was wearing the uniform of the Auxiliary Nursing Service of India and she told me she was on her way home from Burma. "I should be home in just two hours," she said, hardly able to conceal her excitement.

The other woman was still snoring loudly and Margaret told me she was a high caste Hindu woman on her way to Bombay. "She can't speak a word of English," Margaret told me, "so unless your Hindustani is very good you won't be very talkative traveling companions."

As I dressed, I asked Margaret if she knew how one could get to Secunderabad on this line, but she did not know. I told her about Major Stanton and his pathetic attempts at organization and she laughed.

"Oh, he is typical," she said. "Ask the guard or someone at the next station, but I hardly think you will be likely to get a connection at Manmod for Secunderabad."

As soon as the train stopped at the next station I left Margaret to order breakfast and set off in search of an official. Being a small station there was no R.T.O. so I buttonholed the station master who was walking pompously along the platform.

He laughed when I asked if I could get a connection for Secunderabad at Manmod, goodness knows why, and went on to explain how I should get there.

"You will have to change at Nagpur," he said. "The Bombay train gets there tomorrow afternoon and from there you can get a Madras train which stops at Hyderabad. From Hyderabad to Secunderabad is only about seven miles, so you will easily get there."

I thanked him and made for the train again. On the way I met an Englishman. He looked as though he might have been in India for about thirty years and should know his way around so I asked him if he knew how to get to Secunderabad. "Yes, change at Kalyan," he said briefly.

I told him the station master had instructed me differently and he said, "These damn fools never know anything."

As I was getting into my compartment, the guard was just passing by so, for good measure, I asked him where I should change for Secunderabad. "Manmod," he replied promptly.

That did it. I tottered into the compartment and sank into a seat wondering who was mad, me or the rest of the population of India. The Hindu woman had, by this time, emerged from her cocoon and was sitting up chewing betel nut and expectorating with amazing accuracy onto the platform.

Margaret introduced us, speaking to me in her pretty, lilting English and to the Hindu woman in Hindustani. During breakfast, which was served on trays in the compartment, I told Margaret what had happened while I had been out of the train. "It is very conflicting," she said sympathetically. "It isn't fair to send you off on these long trips without arranging things better. It is bad enough for us who have been here all our lives. I'll tell you what though, why not go through to Bombay?"

"That's an idea," I said, brightening.

"Go to the military authorities there and tell them how you have been messed about on this journey and they will have to arrange accommodation for you right through to your hospital. Refuse to budge from there until they do," Margaret said sounding as though she might have experienced similar difficulties, as no doubt she had.

I decided to do that and settled down to a long trip in the company of the unresponsive Hindu woman. I was sorry to see Margaret go when we arrived at her hometown. No one else got in with us during the remainder of the day and the compartment was getting hotter, smellier and dirtier every minute. The woman scattered nut shells and other oddments from her numerous refreshments all over the floor, but I could not call in a sweeper at the many stations we stopped at since she could not run the risk of an "untouchable" casting his shadow on her. Her son was traveling on the train and at most stations he came along to see that she was all right. Fortunately he could speak English, so I managed to keep my vocal chords in working order to some extent. At each station I hung out of the window hoping to catch a glimpse of another white face, but I never saw one. It turned much cooler in the evening and I decided to curl up on my bunk with a book soon after dinner. I was very restless and hardly slept at all that night.

Early the next morning we were invaded by four new arrivals who managed to squash in somehow. There was a tall, beautiful Parsee woman, her two children and their *ayah*. Fortunately the Parsee woman could speak English and she was very interesting, so that was a blessing. The train being for Indians only, no accommodation was made for English cooking and, fond as I was of curry and rice, it became very monotonous when served three times a day.

As the day wore on I was getting more and more fed up with my traveling companions, the heat, the smells, and the disgusting state of the floor. During the late afternoon we stopped at Nagpur station and a further crowd of Indian women and children crowded in. I decided then and there that I could stand no more of it. This was the biggest station I had seen for two days and surely, I thought, anything would be better than going on to Bombay with this crowd. So grabbing a couple of coolies, I and my belongings were transferred to the platform.

Leaving the coolies in charge of my baggage I went to look for the R.T.O. It was quite a distance to his office, up a steep ramp, over a bridge and past several refreshment rooms and other buildings peculiar to Indian stations. There was only a young private in the R.T.O.'s office and he did not look particularly bright, but he was English and I could have hugged him.

"Where's the R.T.O.?" I asked.

"He's on number two platform seeing the Madras mail out," he answered in a broad Northumberland accent.

"Do you happen to know how I can get to Secunderabad?" I asked.

"Yes, that's your train, the Madras mail," he said. "If you hurry you might get on it, but I doubt it. It's packed."

Rushing madly back to where my baggage was I told the coolies to hurry after me with it. They piled it on their heads and set off at a running trot after me to number two platform which was jammed with people. The platform seemed to be miles long and every window of the standing train was packed with British soldiers all yelling, "Plenty of room in here, nursie. Come on, hurry up," to a series of whistles and whoops of delight. White women were so rare to these lads that they never hesitated to show their delight at seeing one.

Finding the R.T.O. in that crowd was like looking for a needle in a haystack and time was flying. Only two minutes and the train would be pulling out. In spite of what the soldiers were saying about there being lots of room, there wasn't an inch of space. Suddenly, I saw a warrant officer who had a red band on his arm so I tackled him. I noticed then that the letters on his sleeve were M.P. and not R.T.O., but he was most eager to help me.

"Come with me," he said, "and I'll get a seat for you."

We went to the end coach and there he put me in an empty first-class compartment. The coolies put my baggage in with me and I asked a sweeper to clean the floor which was littered with rubbish of all kinds. I could hardly believe my good fortune. Only a few minutes ago I had been driven nearly frantic in a carriage full of chattering Indians and here I was with a compartment to myself on a train packed with British soldiers.

"You'll be O.K. now," the warrant officer said. "Change at Hyderabad at three o'clock tomorrow morning."

He saluted smartly and strode off. I tossed a few *annas* to the coolies and the sweeper who were chattering and gesticulating wildly and pointing up the platform. I took no notice of them, but removed my hat and shoes and settled back to enjoy my solitude.

"Where are you going," a respectful Indian voice asked a few seconds later.

I looked down toward the platform and saw a white-uniformed official standing there. "To Secunderabad," I said sweetly, feeling at peace with the world.

"But not on this train," he said.

"Oh, yes I am," I said firmly, wishing he would go away and the train would start moving. "That is, I am going as far as Hyderabad on it."

"But look madam. It is impossible," he said, pointing wildly up the platform, just as the coolies were still doing.

Thinking it might be wise to humor the old fool, I got up and looked out of the window in the direction in which he was pointing, and I got the shock of my life. The remainder of the train had disappeared and I was isolated in my single coach on the end of that great, long platform.

"Well, that's that," I said, feeling as though the end of the world had come. "Where do we go from here?"

I climbed down and motioned to the coolies to get my baggage out again. The sweeper took to his heels, no doubt thinking that I might demand my two *annas* back. The official led the way across the railway lines to the rest rooms where he said I could leave my baggage, have a shower, then see the R.T.O. later about my next move.

"There is another train at half past ten tonight and he might get you on it," he said. "It's a military train."

I thanked him and went inside where I had a most welcome bath and put on a clean battleblouse and skirt. An *ayah* cleaned my shoes and, feeling like a different person, I set off once more for the R.T.O.'s office.

Sitting in his office was a young, fresh-faced lieutenant who seemed delighted to have someone from home to talk to. I gave him a detailed account of my experiences since leaving Ramgarh and after listening sympathetically he promised to do all in his power to get me on the Madras train that night. "I know perfectly well that every berth is booked but I'll do all I can," he said.

I asked him if he knew where I could go for a good dinner and he said if I cared to wait about half an hour he would be happy to take me out to his mess for dinner. I accepted gratefully and while I was waiting conjured up visions of the good English dinner I might get. How welcome it would be after all the curry and rice I had consumed between Tatanagur and Nagpur.

It was a pleasant drive out to the lieutenant's quarters and all the officers there made me feel very welcome.

"Jolly glad to have you," the mess officer said cordially. "In fact it's an honor. We don't get many English girls out here, you know. By the way, we have curry and rice on tonight. I hope you like it."

Forcing a smile, I said there was nothing I would like more.

It was only a quarter after nine when we got back to the station so, taking the R.T.O.'s advice, I went along to the rest room to lie down for an hour.

When I returned to the office, the young private was there again all alone and he informed me that the Madras train would be at least ninety minutes late. Actually, it was nearly four hours late and I was almost speechless with fatigue when it arrived. I was sitting on one of my trunks surrounded by recumbent coolies who were snoring their heads off.

A few minutes after the train pulled into the station the R.T.O. dashed up and said the only berth on the train that was not occupied was in the hospital coach and asked if I would take it. I said I would be glad to. It was a four berth coach and the unoccupied one was an upper berth. The two lower berths were occupied by an elderly Indian doctor and an Anglo-Indian woman doctor. The two of them seemed very annoyed about having their rest disturbed at such an hour and I could see their point, but the third occupant, a R.A.F. officer, climbed down from his upper berth and helped me spread out my bedding roll.

I did not sleep much that night in spite of the fact that I was so tired. The Indian doctor was suffering from acute catarrh and he made disgusting noises all night. The R.A.F. officer coughed violently, but smothered it as well as he could. It sounded like tuberculosis to me and a wave of pity swept through me. No doubt he was yet another victim of a Japanese prison camp.

Since the train was running so late we did not stop for breakfast. The Indian doctor assured me I would have to change at Kazipet and that from there I would be able to get a train to Secunderabad.

Eventually we reached Kazipet and I felt like sending a telegram to Major Stanton to assure him that there really was such a place even though it was not as accessible as he seemed to think, and that I was thirty-six hours behind his schedule.

At Kazipet I fortified myself with a huge meal, after which I found that the Secunderabad train was in the station. The journey from there was a short one, about three hours, and I had delightful traveling companions. I was mentally composing letters I would send to the girls and wondered what it would be like at the new hospital and if I would find anyone there whom I knew.

So I came to Secunderabad. There was a big, well laid out station with attractive shops in the arcades. I made my way to the R.T.O.'s office and asked the sergeant in charge to telephone the military hospital to send a conveyance for me.

I watched him pick up the telephone and then wandered outside to look around and wait for my conveyance. There were only a few days left until Christmas and I was in a strange city where I knew no one, but I was not downhearted. A feeling of excitement gripped me and I was prepared for whatever Secunderabad might have to offer. What I could see of the city looked fresh and green after the heat and glare of the jungle around Ramgarh. I felt, somehow, that I was going to like Secunderabad.

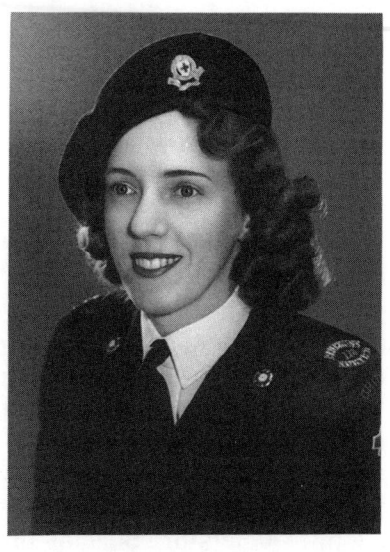

Portrait of Eve in Secunderabad

Chapter Ten

The distance from Secunderabad to Trimulgherry, where the hospital was situated, was about five miles. The transport, when it arrived, proved to be a fifteen hundredweight truck with four Indian soldiers squashed into the front seat. I made them pile my baggage into the back and sat beside the driver, while the other three Indians sat on my trunks.

It was a pleasant drive and the driver pointed out the hospital wards and administrative offices as we passed. The buildings were very scattered and three main roads went through the huge hospital compound. The wards were pink-washed, two-story buildings with high, attractive, arched verandahs and were situated north of the Secunderabad-Trimulgherry Road. South of this road was the sisters' mess, a long, single story building built in a slight hollow.

I alighted from the truck and made my way into the mess to introduce myself to the sister in charge. Her name was Murighy and she was very charming but quite puzzled. She had not heard of the C.M.H., Ramgarh, Major Stanton or me, so obviously they had not been crying out for my services. In fact, I could have been murdered on the train and no one would have been any wiser for perhaps months.

Tea was just being served so we had it together, during which time I was introduced to various members of the mess as they came in for tea. I fell in love with the mess as soon as I saw it. It was the most tastefully furnished and the most spacious mess that I had been a member of since arriving in India. Apparently there were sixty-five of us on the nursing staff.

After tea, Sister Murighy took me up to the bungalows. Being the old Royal Artillery married quarters, they too were the best I had seen. There was not an empty bungalow for me so I had to move in with Mrs. Roberts who was leaving on December 27. Mrs. Roberts was a kindhearted girl from Yorkshire who had been in India only about four months. She made room for me in the three-roomed bungalow and made me feel very welcome.

Mrs. Roberts had gone out so, that night after dinner, I felt tired and very lonely. I crawled into my bed on the verandah feeling very sorry for myself. It was almost Christmas, the first peacetime Christmas since 1938, and I had looked forward to it so much all through those years. I think I might have shed a few tears in self-pity. I am not sure.

I reported to the matron's office next morning for duty and she told me, bless her heart, that I could have the day off to unpack and settle in, so off I skipped. When Mrs. Roberts came off duty she took me into Secunderabad by taxi to show me around and we had tea at the Secunderabad Club. Later, I walked down to the bazaar in Trimulgherry and hired a bicycle.

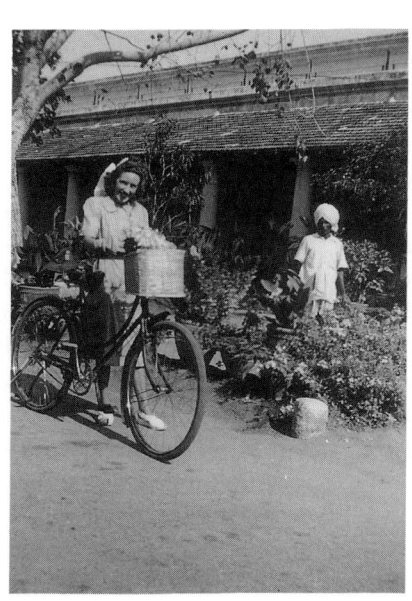

Eve and Mali, the gardener

I was settling down to another quiet evening to write letters when my next door neighbor, a lively Irish girl named Claire Patrick, came in to ask if I would go to a celebration in the medical officers' mess, so I got into evening dress and went along. It was a delightful gathering. Many of the medical officers were Indians and their wives wore some exquisite saris. I was partnered by an R.A.F. officer who drank too much and made a fool of himself. That rather spoiled things for me. Claire was most apologetic about it and introduced me to one of the British doctors who was unattached so I danced with him several times while the R.A.F. character went to put his head under a tap (I hoped).

The next day I was assigned to duty in the mess. There were four of us working there making elaborate preparations for Christmas. It seemed that we were going all out to make this a wonderful Christmas for everyone and I began to get the festive spirit myself. We decorated a huge tree and shopped in the market. Twelve healthy looking turkeys strutted about in the sunshine apparently unaware of the shadow of death hanging over them. The servants, army boys mainly, except for a few civilians, although not Christians were just as excited as we were.

One of the girls in the mess and I went out on our bicycles scrounging flowers and greens from neighboring messes, then we came back and made the mess look almost like a flower show.

They were a gay crowd of girls in the mess and I began to get to know and like them. I even found four girls who had come out on the same ship with me, but they, along with Mrs. Roberts, were being transferred to Madras on December 27.

It was after nine o'clock when I came off duty that night and I was tired but very happy and excited. It looked as though the first peacetime Christmas was going to be the real McCoy.

It was a dark, uphill road from the mess to the bungalows and as I was peddling up on my bicycle, I noticed outlined against the skyline, a car without lights. Wondering what idiot could have parked a car there in the narrow path immediately outside the gates without lights, I decided the safest thing would be to get off my bicycle and wheel it. This I did but a couple of seconds later I found myself falling heavily into the barbed wire entanglement outside the gates, with the bicycle on top of me.

I found it impossible to move or to scramble out as the cruel wire was cutting and scratching me, and anyway I was too dazed. I must have called out as I fell though because the lights of the car were immediately flashed on and I heard excited voices chattering in Hindustani. I felt the bicycle being lifted off me and then tender hands lifted me out.

Still feeling dazed I found that my rescuers were an Indian taxi driver and the white-bearded, dirty-turbaned *chowkidar* did not have the presence of mind to reprimand the driver for parking in such a dangerous spot without lights. Still shaking in every limb, I assured them I was all right and made my way toward the bungalows. I wheeled my bicycle along the verandah and was about to enter my bungalow when Claire's voice called from next door, "Eve, is that you? Come in here a minute will you?"

Anxious for sympathy and human contact, and by now suspicious about a warm sticky trickle down my left leg, I went to the doorway of her bungalow. "I've just made a pot of tea," she began and stopped short. "Why! God love you. You've hurt yourself," she gasped.

I realized then that I had. She put me into a chair and, producing antiseptic and cotton-wool, began swabbing my wounds. There were two long, deep gashes in my left leg and several other minor cuts and bruises all over my arms and legs. Haltingly, I told her about the car and how I had for the moment forgotten about the barbed wire at the gates.

She was furious as she dabbed busily and efficiently at my wounds. As soon as the bleeding was arrested, she gave me a cup of tea and went off on her bicycle to the nearest ward for dressings, still muttering about "stupid Indians who should never be allowed behind the wheel of anything."

It was some time before she returned and when she did she was accompanied by Sister O'Reardon whom she had met on the way. Together they had gone in search of the taxi driver and, both of the girls being Irish, had lashed him with their tongues in no uncertain manner.

Of course the matron had to be told, and I had visions of spending Christmas as a patient in the hospital, but she promised me that as long as the wounds remained clean and since it was Christmas, I didn't need to be confined to bed. I had to report to ward eight twice a day to have my leg dressed and at the first sign of infection I was to be whisked into bed, she said. Fortunately, thanks to my remarkably good health, the wounds never became infected and I was given jobs where I could sit down in the mess with my leg propped up on a chair.

The morning of Christmas Eve my leg was dressed for me by a quiet, shy sister called Pat Collins who asked if I had any plans for the evening. She told me that a young officer in her fiancé's mess had asked her if she knew a girl whom he could take out on Christmas Eve.

"I know it is almost asking the impossible," she said, "but I thought with you being new here you might not know many people yet and would perhaps go with him. He seems a very charming boy."

I said that I had not arranged to do anything that night but with my leg I would not be much fun and, anyway, I was not keen on blind dates. She said she would bring him along for tea in our mess that afternoon so I could meet him, and I agreed to that.

I was doing the accounts in the mess sister's office that afternoon when Pat knocked on the door and said that Robert, her fiancé, and his friend were on the verandah having tea and would I care to join them. I went outside and was introduced. Pat's fiancé looked like the answer to any maiden's prayer, but his companion did not impress me at all. He was of medium height with a very pink, boyish face and looked terribly hot and crumpled. He had what I suspect was the beginning of a military mustache, but I doubted if it would ever amount to anything. Taking his pipe from his mouth he stood up and shook hands with me. I had already decided that I would rather stay home alone than go out with him and wondered how I should word my refusal. The four of us sat down and had tea together, Robert keeping up most of the conversation and my proposed escort contributing very little toward it.

Soon, as I had known it would, the conversation steered round to what I was doing that evening and I said as tactfully as I could that I had no intention of spoiling anyone's Christmas Eve. "I would hardly be the life and soul of any party, would I?" I asked, pointing to the substantial dressing on my left leg.

Neville looked so disappointed that I felt terribly mean. I had visions of the kind of home he came from. Maybe he came from a jolly family like mine and was missing them so much. Knowing how difficult it was for the hundreds of British men in India to get to know girls from home at all, I also thought of the Christmas Eve he would have to spend. In all probability he would drink himself into a stupor in a lonely mess, thinking longingly of home. My conscience bothered me. After all, I thought, it would not hurt me to go out with him just this once. We were both English and six thousand miles from home.

He called at my bungalow for me soon after eight o'clock that night and, as the evenings at this time of the year were quite chilly, he was wearing his serge uniform. As he stepped into the light of the bungalow, I was pleased to see that he was considerably improved in appearance from the hot, dusty young man of the afternoon. He was in fact quite handsome and I think he must have noticed an improvement in me, too. Anyway, he looked approvingly at my full-skirted white evening gown, which fortunately hid the bandages, and told me I looked very sweet.

We saw Pat and Robert as we were getting into our taxi and I was surprised to find they were not joining us, but they were going into Hyderabad to have dinner with an Indian professor whom they knew at the university there. So Neville and I went to the Bolarum Club together.

I guessed that Neville must have been doing a spot of bragging in his mess about having got a date with a girl because some of his unattached fellow officers turned up in full force and he found himself very popular—and so did I. I had dinner with six of them. There was a charming captain called George, but whom everyone called David because of his uncanny resemblance to David Niven. There was also a quiet, clever young major called John, two Scots looking very handsome in their kilts, and a fair-haired recently commissioned cherub called Brian. They were a hilarious bunch. We really got into the spirit of Christmas and I was so glad that I had decided to come. The dining room was a picture and a credit to whoever had hung the decorations. The tables had sunken lamps which set up a soft, flattering light through the leaves and flowers festooning them.

After a delicious dinner and a glass of wine, I decided to try to dance on my injured leg. It was a slow fox trot which I tried with Neville first, and I did quite well. He was an excellent dancer and guided me so skillfully that I did not need to make any quick turns on my left leg.

Christmas Day was hectic for us. The matron had appealed to us to give as much time as possible to the entertainment of the British patients and there was a wonderful response to her appeal. We were kept very busy in the mess during the morning. A crowd of British convalescent patients came over to finish hanging the decorations. Several doctors, British and Indian, dropped in to wish us the compliments of the season. We had a very light lunch and later in the afternoon as many of us as possibly could went to have tea on the British Other Ranks ward. There we danced to a record player. All the beds had been moved along the walls or on the verandahs and I noticed the matron dancing with great enjoyment with a tall, young corporal with only one arm.

We had a real English Christmas dinner in the mess that night and during dinner we heard the king's speech from home. The waiters poured brandy on the Christmas puddings and set them alight. Then they ran between the tables carrying the blazing puddings like excited children. The matron had, out of her own pocket, bought and wrapped presents for all sixty-five of us and after dinner she took them, one by one, off the tree and handed them all to us. As soon as our dinners had digested sufficiently to make walking possible again, most of us went over to the B.O.R. ward again, where we danced until midnight.

The following night we had our big Christmas dance in the mess. We worked hard all day and our efforts were well worth the results. As soon as I could, I went up to my bungalow to bathe and to dress. Neville and John arrived about half past eight and as we walked down the hill we were able to drink in the beauty of the place. The trees in the garden had been hung with tiny colored lights, and tables and chairs were spread out in the garden and on the verandahs. The matron, looking regal in a dark blue evening gown, stood at the top of the steps and was introduced to all our escorts as they arrived. We walked through the dining area where the buffet supper had been set out to join Pat and Robert at a table on the far side of the garden. Robert, who was a keen student of astronomy, told us more that night about the stars than we had ever heard before and it was fascinating.

Two days later there was an afternoon party in the mess and again Robert and Neville were invited. It was supposed to finish at six o'clock but Robert and Neville were still there at nine o'clock as Neville had been persuaded to play the piano and we all joined in a singsong. I was surprised to find that Neville was a brilliant pianist. He played many classics for us. I told him he was a brilliant pianist to which he emphatically replied, "I am not a pianist, I'm an organist."

The following Sunday there were cocktail parties in our mess and in Neville's mess so it was a tossup which of them we should attend. Finally we went to Neville's mess because he said it was time I found out how the poor lived in India. He was always comparing the luxury of our mess with the spartan quarters he lived in.

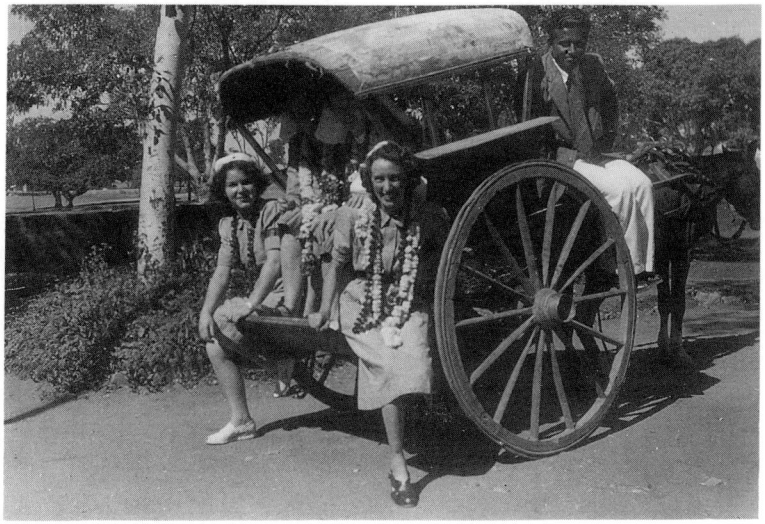

Christmas morning in peacetime, 1945

Chapter Eleven

So the New Year, 1946, came and with it the hottest season of the year. I was transferred to ward six, a busy surgical ward where we were kept very busy with operations. We had several repatriated soldiers from Japanese prison camps, many with broken bones dating back from 1942. Some miraculous bone grafting operations were carried out there.

Late in January there was a bubonic plague scare. A patient in ward five showed all the symptoms of bubonic plague so the whole compound was in quarantine. No one was allowed in or out and we all had to have injections. We obediently presented ourselves for the injections. Ugh! I still shudder when I think of the effect. It was without exception the worst injection any of us had experienced. Within a few hours of the injection we had all the symptoms of plague. Egg-like glands in our groins, necks, and armpits made us a living mass of pain, and temperatures soared. Many doctors and nurses passed out completely, so we found ourselves alarmingly short-staffed in the wards and those of us who were still on duty felt like death. At the end of the week we were supposed to report for a second injection but by that time the patient who was supposed to have the plague was found to be negative, so the hospital was back in circulation and very few of us had the second injection after all.

Gradually many of the men we knew were being sent home for demobilization. That, more than anything, made us realize that the war was really over and everyone began to get restless. Life went on as usual in the mess with many little incidents important to us but of little or no interest to the outside world. Dr. Kenny's wife who worked on ward eight found that she was going to have a baby so she was packed off to

England. Dr. Meadows married Sister Grant and the matron gave them a wonderful reception in the mess. Sister Bell married an army officer from Bombay. There were several engagements, a few broken ones, Verna Frances had a tonsillectomy and one of the nurses was in a car crash in which she was the only survivor.

Joan Harcourt-Dell created a minor scandal and, after a severe reprimand from the matron, set off to hitchhike to Palestine to join her husband who was there. However, she only got as far as New Delhi. She was intercepted there, sent back to us and was then sent to England. Actually, she went to the transit camp in Deolali, hid her discharge papers in her luggage and took a civilian post right there in the transit camp. She was not discovered until several months later and that was only because Dr. Meadows passed through the transit camp on his way home to England and saw her working in the general office there. That was the end of her capers. She really was packed off to England then.

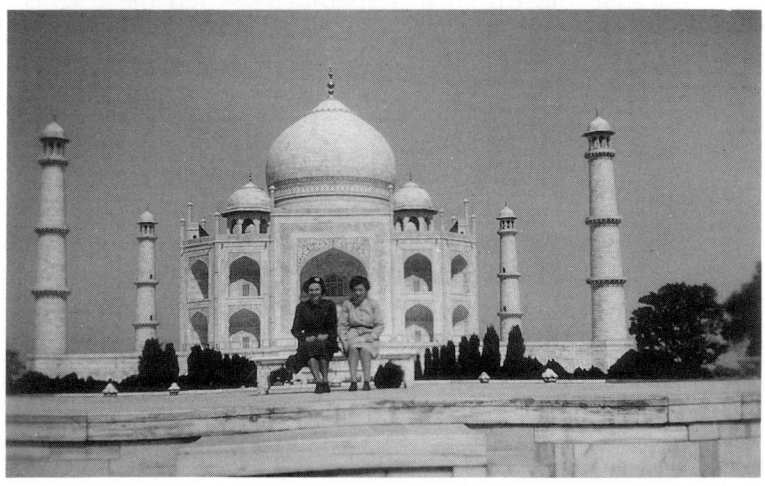

The Taj Mahal, Agra

In February I met Elizabeth, my Canadian friend, again. She was still stationed in Chhindwara, so we met in New Delhi and then went to Agra together to see the Taj Mahal. There was great excitement when General Auchinleck visited the hospital and decorated one of the sisters. She was awarded the Medal of the British Empire (M.B.E.) in the New Year's honors list for quelling a riot in her ward the previous year. A fight had broken out between some Indian patients under her care. A Sikh was stabbed and another one was about to be stabbed when Penny calmly sailed in and twisted the attacker's arm until he dropped the knife. Her ward boy picked up the knife and ran for help. The Sikh died, three of the patients were put in detention and what might have been a very bad Hindu-Moslem riot was averted because of Penny's quick action.

About this time I went on night duty again and became friendly with Marie Bentley, the night sister in charge. Neither of us had visited Ootacammund so we decided to go there on leave together as soon as we could.

Many of the British troops had moved out of the area since Christmas and it had been rumored for some time, and then became a fact, that we had to vacate the hospital premises in April because the Nizam of Hyderabad wanted the premises for his own state troops, no doubt to help quell the Hindu-Moslem riots which were getting worse all over India.

After night duty I was transferred back to day duty in the mess. Sister Murighy had asked the matron if she could have me back there to help her in the mess because a short spell with Delia Martin had nearly driven her frantic. Besides, all the mess furniture and equipment had to be catalogued and packed as well as the accounts had to be balanced and paid. Being in part-British, part-Indian territory, we had two currencies to cope with and poor Murighy had no head for figures. So I had to do the accounts, assisted by our gorgeous butler, Dina. Dina was a tall, imposing-looking Hindu and a disgusting snob. He considered it much beneath his dignity to be a butler for a bunch of nurses after working for a British general for fifteen years. The general had retired to England and as the British were gradually leaving India anyway, Dina could not be as choosy about his jobs as he had been in the past.

I could understand why Sister Murighy wanted to get rid of Delia Martin, because she was the despair of most of us.

Everyone was of the opinion that she was crazy, but I will be more charitable and say that the Indian sun seemed to be having the worst possible effect on her. She was supposed to be the widow of a R.A.F. man but Neville said it was his belief that the poor fellow was hiding from her. Her main objectives in life were apparently to find another husband and to decipher her bank account.

Even in India where men were ten a penny, they shied away from poor Delia. She was frequently seen at the clubs unaccompanied, an unheard of thing. I had often seen her cycling along the Bolarum Road in something outlandish—a swimsuit, evening dress, and even pajamas. Periodically she would be packed off to hospital for observation and complete rest, but even there, when no one was around she would sneak off to go out to dances.

Delia's finances seemed to be as strained as her health and tradesmen hounded her at every step, flourishing checks which had bounced.

"My family has banked with Lloyd's for generations," she would moan, "but I shall never trust them again. Whenever I write a check they refuse to cash it."

"Naturally," I would say, "when there are no funds to meet it," but she would look at me as though she thought I must be as unscrupulous as Lloyds Bank.

The last straw was one night at a fancy dress ball at the Bolarum Club. She had frantically canvassed the mess to find someone who had a spare man, but no one would bite. I felt very guilty when she approached me because I was going with Neville and John, but they would have lynched me had I asked her to join us, so I said that as far as I knew I was only going with Neville. It looked as though she would not be able to go but she did. She went alone and was sitting on the club verandah when I arrived with my two escorts. What she was supposed to be dressed as no one seemed to know. I said possibly Bo-Peep, and Neville said she looked like a Dresden shepherdess. John said she looked like the Dame in the last pantomime he saw but he never explained.

She wore a pale blue silk gown with a full skirt. It had three-quarter length lace sleeves and for reasons best known to her, she had tacked a lace doily across the back of the dress. She wore a black felt pillbox hat and a black domino. She tried very hard to join our party but the boys would have none of it and she finally ran down a gin-soaked major who was also something of an outcast. The next day she was packed off to a hospital several miles away for a "complete rest." I sincerely hope she got it because she was certainly in need of it.

Several nurses shared a delightful servant who was not only a good, honest worker, but could speak excellent English. In February he was to be married and he invited some of us to the wedding reception. He came into my bungalow one evening and, grinning from ear to ear, handed me a printed invitation. There were four pages of it and, fortunately, one of them was in English. Briefly, it told me that Madurai Pillay and Andal Ammall would be married on February 11, 1946. The dinner following the long ceremony would be at 10 P.M. at Lingham Street, Ammaguda and there would be music. Never having been to an Indian wedding celebration, I certainly was anxious to go. He looked pleased when I said I would be happy to go and then asked if I would bring "English officer sahibs" too. I knew, of course, why he would want British army officers there. He would be able to lord it over his neighbors forevermore.

Politely I wished him many blessings and much happiness. I said I was sure she must be a very nice girl. "Oh, yes, memsahib," he assured me adding that he was sure his parents had selected a most suitable bride for him. It was apparent that he had never met her, which was customary until the day of the wedding.

As further encouragement to bring as many officer sahibs as I could, he promised that we would be served good English *khana* (food). I wondered apprehensively what that might consist of.

Madurai was a good servant so the nurses put their heads together, and in accordance with his wishes, we scouted around among the doctors and the neighboring messes for men who would like to attend. As hardly any of them had been to an Indian wedding reception either, every man asked was anxious to go.

February, still being winter and, therefore, quite cold in the evenings, we all decided to wear our dress uniforms instead of the usual drab khaki. That would really impress the neighbors!

We were a good-sized crowd, all of us shining from spit and polish. Shoes and Sam Brown belts shone like mahogany and brass buttons shone like gold, shirts were fresh from our *dhobi wallahs* (washermen) and all hats were at the correct angle. We would have done credit to any parade. The place was teeming with Indians when we got there, many of them inebriated, and all thronged around us greeting us with smiles and the Indian greeting of hands raised, palms together and head slightly bowed.

The sixteen-year-old bride, wearing a bright orange sari, looked scared and shy. A small fortune must have been spent on the wonderful array of food. There were delicious curries of all kinds, great dishes of saffron rice, bowls of tempting food and nuts that always accompany curries. Over to the side were what looked like mountains of the colorful and sweet desserts which Indians love. Our mouths watered. To heck with the good English *khana* we all thought.

Madurai's father, a small man with a nut-brown wrinkled face, steered us away from the groaning tables and bowed us out to the garden.

"Please come," he said. "We just now ready to serve you good English *khana*. Outside, please. You come."

There was nothing else to do. With a longing look at the tempting food, we followed him into the garden. It was a very small garden, not really big enough for the big table which had been prepared for us. The table was covered with white sheets and several places set. It was lit by candles in gourds.

At each place setting was a knife, fork, spoon, glass, cup and saucer. In the center of the table were teapots and bottles of whiskey. Between each knife and fork was a plate of rather sad looking fish and chips. With aching hearts, we thanked them profusely for the "wonderful spread." So much for their ideas of English food. Was this all we had impressed upon them during the many years of British raj?

There was a cockroach on one of the plates of fish and chips that put us all off completely. How thankful we were that our table was outdoors, that it was fairly dark and there were hungry *pai* dogs around.

About this time, Hyderabad was out of bounds to us for a short time. Bombay and Calcutta had on occasions been out of bounds to British troops not there on urgent business because of the Hindu-Moslem riots, but this was the first time that Hyderabad had been subjected to a big riot. The town hall was burned down and the mayor had his mustache cut off by incensed rioters. It seemed to me that they were making more fuss than was necessary about the mayor's mustache and I said so to Dina, our butler.

"It was a raggy old mustache anyway," I said, "and he certainly looks much better without it." A pained expression crossed Dina's face as he tried to explain to me the magnitude of such a heinous offense.

"No Hindu ever shaves his mustache during the lifetime of his father," he said in sepulchral tones.

Ah, well, one lives and learns.

Chapter Twelve

A major catastrophe occurred in late March. Neville and his colleagues were posted to Northern Command. We had by this time become great friends and I hated to see him go, but that was the way things always were in the army.

Life seemed very dull after he left and when a fresh batch of nurses arrived I once again found myself sharing a bungalow with another person. The newcomer was named Belinda Carruthers and could not possibly have been more different from me if she had tried. My neat and tidy bungalow took on the appearance of a secondhand shop. Drawers were permanently open with odds and ends of clothing spilled over the sides, dirty clothing lay on the floor awaiting the *dhobi wallah*, cigarette ends littered every inch of space and dresses were anywhere except in the wardrobes.

Belinda smoked like a chimney and drank like a fish. Her constant cry seemed to be, "I must have a little tipple," and she would get out a bottle of gin if it were before noon and a bottle of Scotch if it were later. She could drink spirits like a man, yet I never saw her drunk.

At first having to live amidst such untidiness worried me but as she said, "Listen, kid, if I don't let your tidiness get on my nerves, you mustn't let my untidiness get on yours." So we made the best of each other. It seems incredible that although we were so different in every way we got along so well together. I always disapproved of her intemperance and her questionable morals but I took off my hat to her kindness. She was a slave to duty and worried about many of her patients who all adored her.

One evening as she sat in the bungalow pensively sipping a Scotch and soda, I could see that she was worried about something but I did not say anything or force her confidence as I knew that she would tell me in her own time.

"You know, Eve, the Indians are funny people," she said eventually. "There's going to be trouble here, soon too. I am going to sleep indoors and bolt all the doors and windows."

"Why?" I asked. "Are you afraid the pink elephants in green spats will come to get you?"

She smiled faintly. "Don't worry, kid. I haven't got D.T.'s yet," she said. "But I am worried about the political and religious situation here, and now that I have seen what they can think up to do to people," she shuddered.

"Why? What have you seen?" I asked.

"Have you seen Saki?"

I said no, but I had heard about him. Saki was a patient in Belinda's ward who had been badly burned with acid several months before.

"You ought to see him," she said. "Everyone ought to see him. He is the living proof of how cruel and vindictive these people can be."

I asked what on earth she was talking about because as far as I knew Saki's face had been burned in an accident.

"Accident my foot!" Belinda burst out. "He told me all about it today. He was sleeping peacefully when a colleague who was jealous of him poured acid on his face."

"Oh, no!" I shuddered. "What was he jealous of?"

"He was jealous because Saki had passed an exam which he had failed, so you see what I mean about these people. They are so cruel and cunning. If they can hate their own people as much as that, think how much more they must hate the British now that they want to govern themselves. Who is to say what might happen to us when we are sleeping out there on the verandah? Not me. I'm sleeping in here. I shall ask Hussain to move my bed at once." She dashed out into the night and called loudly for the servant.

It was the first time I had seen the placid Belinda so upset but I made no comment when Hussain came in and pulled her bed inside. I knew what was really the matter was that she had become consumed with pity for the poor, unfortunate boy with no face. She told me later that he had shown great promise and had a brilliant future ahead of him in the Indian Navy, but all that was lost now.

"I must do something for him," she moaned, "but what can I do?"

I suggested that she should take him for a walk occasionally and she seemed to think that was a good idea.

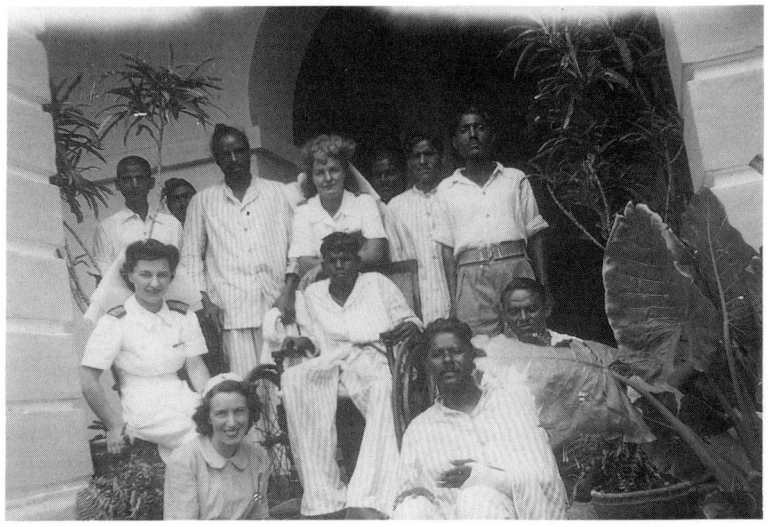

The nurses and their patients

"By jove, I will," she said. "You know he just lies there; can't read Braille or anything and no one bothers to take him anywhere, yet he is quite fit physically. I can take him outdoors and lead him by the hand. It will certainly give him a new interest in life even if he can't see anything."

That was how it was in the weeks that followed: a familiar sight to be witnessed around the hospital compound was a slight Indian boy with no eyes and a mass of charred flesh where his face had once been, hanging trustingly on the arm of tall, blond Belinda.

At the beginning of April the mess was buzzing with excitement. Four of the sisters, Edwards, Jones, Burrill, and Patrick were going home. No one really begrudged them their good luck because, after all, they had served in India longer than any of us and Burrill and Patrick especially were beginning to show the strain of hard work and cruel climate. It was my half day off and I knew it would be Claire's too, so as I cycled up the hill I wondered if she would like to go to the club for a swim.

As I wheeled my bicycle along the verandah I could see into her bungalow. Already she was dismantling it and with a pang I realized how much I would miss my kind next door neighbor with her numerous cups of tea and her Irish brogue. Cycling up the hill was so exhausting and I was glad to step into her cool, shaded bungalow, where the electric fan whirring overhead was a welcome sound.

"Going somewhere?" I asked, flopping into the nearest chair and taking stock of the scattered garments and open trunks, at one of which she was kneeling.

"Haven't you heard?" she asked wide eyed. "I'm going home for demobilization."

"Yes, I've heard," I replied. "You lucky dog. Don't forget to give my love to Blighty."

"To be sure, I will," she promised. "Do you know I can't tell whether 'tis my head or my feet I'm on. I'm so excited; you have no idea."

"I'm sure you must be," I said. "Gosh, Claire, it must be a wonderful feeling. I just can't imagine it. I've been trying to, but somehow it seems impossible."

"I know. Many's the time I have tried to imagine what it would be like to really know you were going home, but I never could." Her face had a faraway look but suddenly it broke into a smile. "Don't worry, darling your turn will come," she said. "This is the start."

"Seems funny to think of the war being over, doesn't it?" I asked. "Nearly a year of peace, but we haven't really found much difference here. Imagine seeing Piccadilly and Leicester Square with lights again. I can't remember how they looked with them, you know."

"Well it won't be long now before you will see it all again," Claire said with confidence. "I only hope we shall find that brave new world they have promised us. Think of that glorious long leave and those postwar credits."

"Would you like to go for a swim this afternoon?" I asked her.

"I'll have to pack. I have no time to go swimming," she said. "Then I'm going down to see Nabi Bux to get some presents to take home."

"Good heavens!" I gasped. "You have a fortnight in which to pack. Besides it's no use packing now. You are too excited."

"That's true, I am," she laughed. "But it's a natural reaction to start packing the minute you hear such startling news—just in case they change their minds, I suppose."

"Got anything worth giving away?" I asked surveying all the things scattered around.

"I'll be throwing all sorts of things out I suppose," she said.

"This is a good pair of monsoon boots," I said reminding her that we both wore the same size and she had seen her last monsoon season.

"You keep your eyes off those boots," she said. "They are going home with me. You can't get boots like that here or at home now and they'll be grand for the winter in Ireland."

"All right, meanie, keep them," I said. "What time are you going to see Nabi Bux?"

"Pretty soon," Claire replied. "Would you like to come with me?"

"No. I can't be bothered," I said, "but I'll cycle as far as the club with you. I'm going for a swim."

Belinda arrived at that moment with Saki. She usually took him for a walk about this time and sometimes called in at the bungalows.

I could see that she was excited about something, so excited in fact that she dashed over the doorstep without waiting to see that Saki could manage.

"Eve, guess what?" she said.

"I don't need to," I said hollowly. "I already know. Claire, Burrill, Jones and Edwards are going home, lucky blighters."

"So are we."

I blinked. "Eh?" I gasped, rudely.

"You and I are going home too. We have to be in Poona on the twenty-eighth of this month," Belinda said slowly.

"Belinda, that is not funny," I said coldly. "No one should joke about anything so sacred."

She laughed. "I'm not joking," she protested. "Honestly, Eve. The matron just sent for us to go to her office, so I went along and told her you had gone off duty for the day. Then she said that word had come through from New Delhi that you and I were due for demobilization and that we are to report to the transit hostel in Poona on the twenty-eighth. From there we shall go to Bombay for a ship."

At last she managed to convince me that she was speaking the truth.

"Claire," I yelled. "You can keep your wretched monsoon boots," and I gave her a bear-like hug.

The three of us were almost weeping with delight, then Belinda remembered Saki who had managed to stride over the threshold and was standing uncertainly in the doorway leaning on the carved stick which the ward sister had given him for his twenty-first birthday and of which he was so proud.

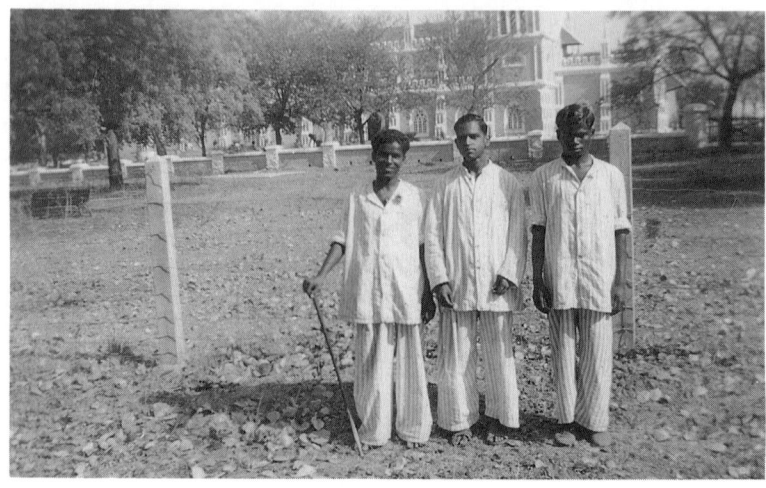

Patients outside Garrison Church in Trimulgherry

"Saki, I'm so sorry," Belinda said, immediately concerned because we had ignored him. She led him to a chair.

"Don't worry about me, Sister," he said in his faultless English. "I know how happy you are to go home to England. I am happy too, because you are, but I shall be very sad when you go. It will be the saddest day of my life."

There was such genuine feeling in his voice that I felt a tightening in my throat. Yes, there was no doubt about it, these boys would miss us. What would happen to them when they were being taken care of by Indian nurses and orderlies? Would they, with their ever prominent caste system and their religious hatreds, be as sympathetic toward them as we had been? I thought of poor nineteen-year-old Ali Mamoud in ward six with his gun-shattered abdomen, Gopal Rai whose throat had been wounded to such an extent that he had to have a permanent tracheotomy in order to make breathing possible. These and many others who had become so dependent on us. As for Saki, I doubt if he would have got around at all if Belinda had not taken him in hand and encouraged him to overcome his dreadful affliction.

I suddenly realized as I looked at Saki, sitting there so forlorn, that we were bound to miss him too. It was easy to forget his affliction when talking to him as he was so clever and interesting. With his education and ambition he would have been sure of a brilliant future in the new India that was to be, but now, well it was hard to guess what would become of him. We were used to seeing the distorted mass of flesh that his face had become, but would his relatives and friends? It was very doubtful and that was why we always covered his whole head with gauze and let it hang down to his shoulders, something like a motoring veil from early motoring days.

Similar thoughts must have entered the minds of Belinda and Claire because they had become very quiet and I thought I saw Claire quickly brush a tear from her cheek. Belinda gave Saki a cigarette and Claire lit it for him. He had somehow mastered the art of holding a cigarette between his perfect teeth as he had no lips.

With the gauze covering drawn back he puffed contentedly at his cigarette and asked which of the nurses were going home. He only needed to hear any of us speak once and he always remembered our voices.

"Perhaps when I come to England for plastic surgery I can visit all of you and show you what a good job the surgeons have done to my face," he said.

"Why of course, Saki," Belinda said. "That would be wonderful. We will come to the hospital to see you."

Saki had great faith in what would eventually be done to his face. He finished his cigarette, Claire gave him an orange, and Belinda said it was time they were getting back to the ward. Neither of us spoke as we watched them walk along the verandah, Belinda matching her steps to his slow uncertain ones. No doubt Claire was thinking the same as I was.

"Come on, Claire," I said when they were out of sight. "I think I might as well go along and see Nabi Bux with you."

Our spirits were bright again as we cycled along the road to Hyderabad. It always gave me a pleased little thrill when I saw the signpost at Percy's corner. It read: "Hyderabad—7.5 miles; London 6,449 miles."

Nabi Bux was not at home when we got there but his son assured us that he would be back shortly. He bowed us inside the small, smelly house and dusted a couple of chairs for us which were kept especially for such visitors. He put cigarettes and an ashtray within easy reach of us and asked if we would like some tea. Not being too confident about his water supply we declined, but so as not to hurt his feelings, we each accepted an orange when he offered them. They were safe enough with their thick, undamaged skins.

We told him we had come to find some good presents at reasonable prices to take to England, so he dragged out the bulk of his father's stock and set it before us. Like Nabi, his son was the essence of politeness and interspersed his remarks with hundreds of "sirs" irrespective of the sex of whoever he was talking to.

Nabi Bux came in not long afterward and by then we had picked out all that we wanted and all that remained was to persuade the old man to let us have them at the prices we wanted to pay. His son was squatting on the floor with six exquisitely hand-embroidered nightgowns and slips spread over his shoulders. We admired them of course, but decided we could not possibly afford them and, anyway, something more durable would be better to take home as souvenirs of India.

Jewelry and carved boxes littered the floor and a couple of Kashmir rugs which I had made up my mind to buy were rolled up beside the door. There was a wonderful carved box which I was dying to take home for Dorothy, but which he seemed determined not to knock down to less than eighty rupees.

"Nabi, be a sport," I implored. "I'll give you thirty-five rupees, but I can't possibly afford any more."

"No, sir," Nabi said firmly. "There is no one I would rather see have that box, but I am giving it away when I ask only eighty rupees."

"Well you can afford to give it away," I said. "You must be rolling in money."

"No, no, sir. Nabi is a very poor man," he whined.

"I'll bet there's only one man richer than you in the whole of Hyderabad," I said, "and that's the Nizam."

Poor Nabi laughed so much I thought his cascade of stomachs would never stop shaking. He enjoyed his laugh so much that he let me have the box for forty rupees, so from that I gathered that it must have been worth at least twenty-five.

With our purchases completed, and Nabi having promised to deliver everything the following day, we got on our bicycles and rode off. Nabi, his son, his servant, and half the neighborhood waved frantically to us until we were out of sight.

Chapter Thirteen

We left Secunderabad on a Sunday—such a strange day of partings and packings. Five of us were going to Poona together, Verna Frances, two Canadian nurses, Vi Kemp and Rae Summers, Belinda and myself. Now that the day had dawned, even though we were returning to England, parting was a wrench. I took a last ride on my hired cycle to visit all the wards and say my good-byes. Some of the patients cried openly, and on ward six, Marie Bentley was bemoaning the fact that our hopes of leave in Ootacamund had been so rudely shattered.

There was a dejected droop to my servant's shoulders as he pottered around my bungalow that morning and I felt sorry for him. Not that he was a good servant—even his best friends could not have said that about Hussain. In fact, there were times when I thought he must be the world's worst. I had tried so often to dismiss him but although he was not a good servant, he was a wonderful psychologist. He seemed to have an uncanny knowledge of it every time I made up my mind to get rid of him once and for all and would appear with something that would put my mind right off it, for the time being anyway.

Frequently, after a hard spell of duty in the hospital, I would return to the bungalow to find my bed unmade, my bathwater not emptied, dirty uniforms still waiting to be given to the *dhobi wallah,* and every piece of furniture coated with the fine white dust that was always everywhere in India. I would be hot, tired and very annoyed. How impatiently I would await Hussain's appearance so that I could fire him once and for all, but with that uncanny instinct of his, when he did appear it would be with a long tale of woe. He may have found the sweeper stealing something from the bungalow and had chased him and beaten him, or maybe one of his children had been gravely injured. He might even appear with a broad grin splitting his brown face in two and holding out a huge bouquet of flowers.

"For you, memsahib," he would say with a sweeping bow. "I just now bring. Many long miles I go for them because I know you like flowers, memsahib." Of course, I knew that he had stolen the flowers, possibly from someone's garden a few yards away, and he knew that I knew it. He also knew that I was too soft to fire him anyway and that I was haunted by the pitiful spectacle of humanity he had been when he first came to work there. He was so sick and emaciated that one wondered how he managed to walk around. But now after a few months, although he was still painfully thin and coughed distressingly, he was looking much better and since his wife and children had been eating regularly, they were in better health.

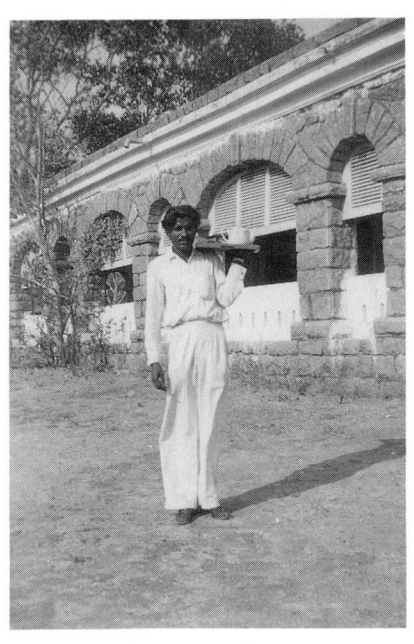

Hussain, Eve's bearer

So I put up with him for as long as I had to. I asked myself how I would like to live on forty rupees a month. And I forgave him for drying my dishes on shoe dusters and using my good teacloths and pillowcases for polishing the furniture. At least I knew it was not forever.

And now I was going home and Hussain was in low spirits. The bungalow looked so strange both to him and to me. Instead of making my bed he had to strip it and make up my bedding roll for the train. There was nothing for him to put away in the drawers. The drawers were empty and the shelves were bare. Even the floor looked unfamiliar without my Kashmir rugs and the burn which Neville's pipe had made on the table was now exposed for the whole world to see, instead of being discreetly hidden by a table mat.

After everything had been packed I sent Hussain to the bazaar to return my bicycle. He was openly crying as he rode off and I felt awful. I wondered if the average Indian wanted to see the end of British rule in India. Would Hussain be hungry again after we had left? Who would employ the millions like him? It all made me feel so depressed. Verna, coming along the verandah at that moment asked me whose funeral I was attending.

"Hussain's," I said flatly.

"Oh! I didn't know he was dead," she said showing interest.

"He isn't, but who will employ him after we move out?" I asked.

"Some mug, I expect," Verna said easily. Verna never lost any sleep over anything.

"But he may be hungry again," I said.

"Not unless he has squandered all those odd *annas* he has pinched from me every time I have sent him shopping," Verna replied. "To say nothing about what he has pinched from all the other girls."

"But Verna," I protested. "I honestly don't think he has ever stolen anything from me."

Verna laughed. "My dear Eve," she said patiently, "even an illiterate Indian would know better than to try and do a Yorkshire woman out of her change."

"Don't be rude," I said. "But seriously though, Verna."

"Listen, kid," she broke in, "it's no use worrying. You might as well say who is going to buy all that junk from the bazaars that the British have been buying for so long. Can you see the Indians buying all those ghastly souvenirs with the Taj Mahal plastered all over them? How many dresses and shoes will be sold? Who isn't going to be hungry? Precious few I can assure you. There's going to be trouble here, soon too. They have brought it all on themselves, and the best thing we can do is to thank our lucky stars that we shall be six thousand miles away."

"It's all so bewildering," I said. "I wish I had studied the whole question more. I have never taken sufficient interest in politics, I know, but I will in the future. Wonder what it will be like at home under a labor government."

"Stinko, I suppose," Verna said. "I refuse to be worried about it at this stage in the proceedings though. I'm going to have a nice little holiday on that old steamer."

The matron and Sister O'Reardon, along with a host of our friends, went to the station to see us off on the train to Poona. Again, accommodations were very cramped. We found that we had been allotted a four-berth coach between the five of us so Vi and Rae volunteered to share a lower berth. Belinda took the other lower berth and Verna and I the two upper ones. Our twenty-two pieces of luggage were duly weighed and checked and it was arranged for most of it to be put in the luggage van.

We stood around on the platform making the usual remarks prior to the departure of a train. Over and over again we were reminded to lock all the doors and windows before we settled down for the night or someone would be sure to climb in and cut our throats.

At last it was time for the train to move so we hung out of the windows waving frantically. The matron was surreptitiously dabbing her eyes and O'Reardon was trying to be ever so cheerful. The train moved slowly down the long platform and we leaned further and further out so that we could see them all as long as possible. It was very touching, but at the very end of the platform we suddenly saw our baggage still standing there. There was an instant of panic and then Vi pulled the communication cord. The train came to a halt and all the coolies got very excited. This looked like fun! An indignant official came up and demanded to know who had pulled the communication cord. Vi, in a few well-chosen words, told him that she had and asked if he would kindly explain what our baggage was doing on the platform when it was supposed to be in the luggage van.

He said we had no right to pull the cord and stop the train without just cause, and we said that we had just cause. Then he gave us the old patter about having to run to schedule. We pointed out that as the train was already fifty-two minutes late, two minutes more to get our stuff on board was neither here nor there. He ordered a crowd of coolies to put the luggage in the luggage van but we told him we had heard enough about his luggage van and we would have it all in the compartment with us. He said it was impossible to get it all in, but we were adamant. We were prepared to put up with the congestion in the compartment for the sake of having everything under our eyes.

By this time all our friends and well-wishers had walked down the platform, so good-byes had to be said all over again and the warnings about homicidal bandits to be repeated. At last we were off, Belinda and I being almost completely cut off from the girls at the other side of the compartment. The toilet was at their side and it was like making an alpine tour over mountains of luggage for us to get there. The journey was only an overnight one and we turned in fairly early. Before doing so we made short work of the hamper which O'Reardon had ordered to be packed for us. There was cold chicken, salad, cake and lots of fruit.

We lay on our berths and talked for a long time after putting the lights out. Vi and Rae made themselves reasonably comfortable by lying at opposite ends of the bunk they were sharing. Finally, one by one, we dropped off to sleep.

It must have been long past midnight when I was awakened by the most horrible bloodcurdling shrieks. My stomach turned over. The shrieks were right in the compartment and were going on and on. I could not make out who was shrieking and switched on the light above me but still could not see much because of the mountain of luggage, but I could see Verna leaning out of her bunk. Belinda, beneath me, was demanding to know who was being hurt, and after a few nasty moments it all came out.

Apparently Vi, in her sleep, had pushed her foot up under Rae's chin. Rae had awakened and felt something at her throat. Thinking she was being strangled, she made a grab for the foot. Vi, waking and feeling something pulling at her foot, had let out a scream of terror. So what with Vi pushing her foot harder and Ray pulling, and neither of them knowing what was going on, they were having a terrific struggle and making an awful din. It was all very nerve-shattering and getting to sleep again proved somewhat difficult. It seemed I was never to have an uneventful journey on an Indian train.

So I came to Poona again. This time we were housed in a hospital on the other side of town, the number three general

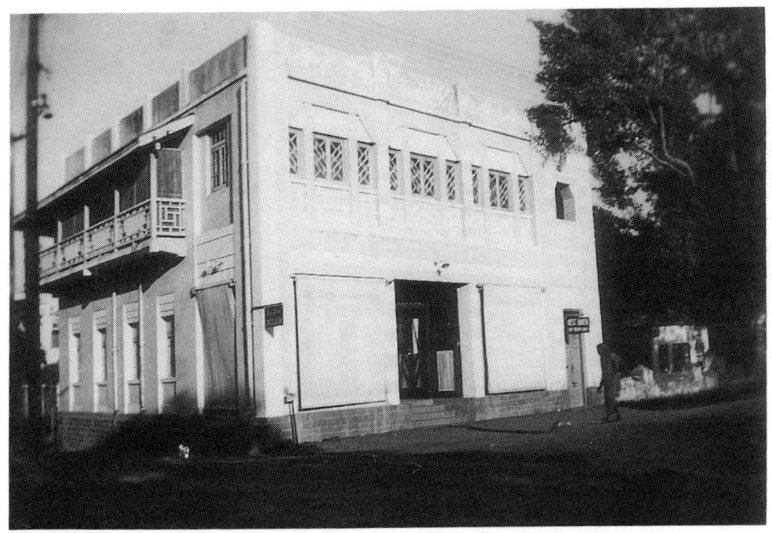

Services Club, Poona

hospital. The British Military Hospital was situated in an adjoining compound and it was often difficult to tell which buildings belonged to which hospital. When we arrived we were taken to a long dormitory and allotted beds in it. Suddenly I saw Elizabeth and nearly fell over in surprise. With a shriek of delight I leapt over the three or four beds separating us and descended upon her. How we talked and talked. She had known I was coming because she had read the list of new arrivals on the notice board. She had arrived the previous day and in her party were two other girls who had come out on the same ship with us. What a joyous reunion we had. Apart from the fact that we were going to see our "ain folk" again, none of us was wildly excited about going home. I think we were all rather dubious about the brave new world we had been fighting for—and then of course there was Sir Stafford Cripps.

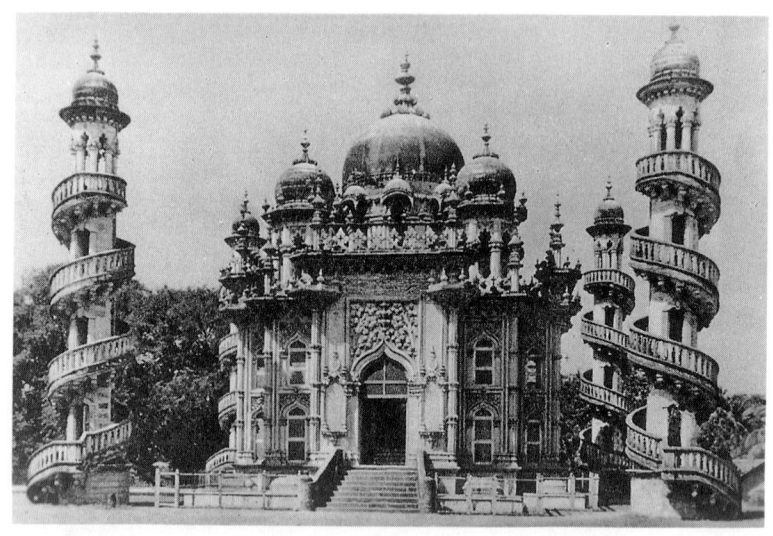

"The Times of India" office

We stayed in Poona for a week and what a lot we crowded into that week. This was our last touch with the great continent of India. We tore around madly buying all the trash we had been planning to buy ever since we arrived, but had never done so. Most of us drained our banking accounts to the dregs. We went to the Poona Club again, but it still seemed to be mourning the loss of its original *pukka* (important) sahibs.

One day I took Belinda to the administrative offices to get her vaccination certificate signed. "I know where it is," I assured her, but unfortunately I took her into the wrong building. I thought we were still in the number three hospital compound but we were not. We were in the British Military

Hospital (BMH) compound and my error was the cause of her having a cholera injection then and there, something which she had always managed to avoid. The next day she had a very bad arm, but managed to see the funny side of it.

"I'm so glad you didn't take me into the operating theater by mistake," she said. "I might have lost a perfectly good appendix or something."

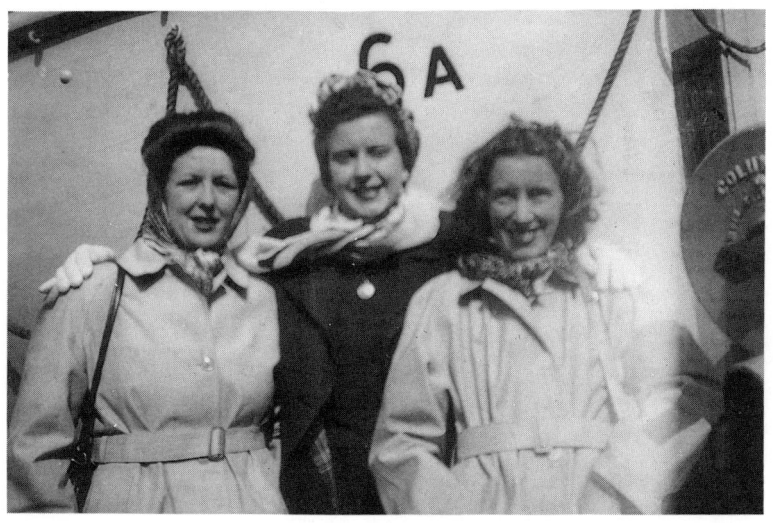

Going Home!

Soon our week in Poona was over and we were lining up on the dockside in Bombay to board the ship. It was a huge ship and every porthole seemed to be jammed with troops' heads. They cheered loudly when we arrived, not that there was anything spectacular about us. Troops just like cheering when they are hanging over the side of a ship. Anyway, they were going home, so they had some excuse for cheering.

I blushed furiously when I handed over the residue of my Indian currency to be converted into sterling. It was hardly worth the trouble, and I was wondering how I would manage on the seventeen-day trip with so little money, but fate smiled on me. Who should be on the ship, having just arrived from Deolali, but dear Mildred? After the preliminary greetings were over, she said, "Say, Eve, I never gave you back the fifteen rupees I borrowed from you in Calcutta, did I?" and she handed me a beautiful crisp pound note and a bright shiny half-crown which I pounced on with glee.

Once on board it was like old home week. There were so many old friends on board I began to wonder if the whole of the British nursing service had been withdrawn together, and, best of all, there was dear Claire, my next door neighbor from Secunderabad.

Altogether there were six thousand people on board so it was not surprising that we met so many whom we had known on our travels through India. There were a few officers from the Royal Engineers we had known in Kalyan, a couple of doctors from Ranchi, and quite a number from Secunderabad, all going home for demobilization.

The ship was overcrowded and uncomfortable, but as I said to Belinda, "The powers that be know perfectly well they don't even have to try to keep up our morale on the way home."

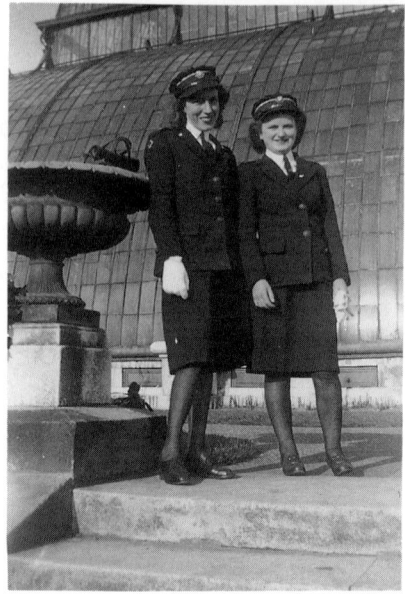

Home again

With a slight feeling of regret I stood and watched Bombay fade into the distance when the great ship pulled out. India, fascinating India, with her heat and smells, her diseases, religions, extreme wealth and extreme poverty had somehow found a place in my heart and I vowed that one day I would return.

Then, after seventeen days at sea, I was home. The ship docked at Liverpool and there was no one at the dockside to greet me but I took a delight in watching other people looking for their relatives and friends. It seemed strange for everyone waiting on the dockside to be white skinned after living among Indians for so long.

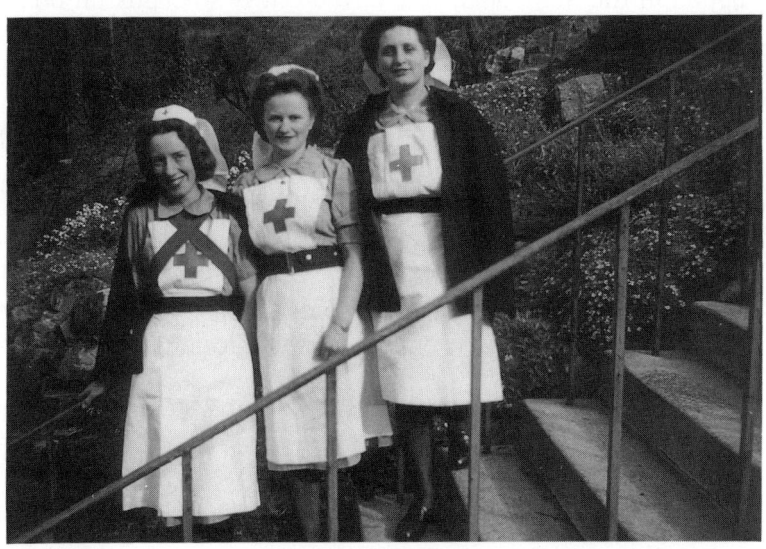

Back on duty in the UK

Verna, whose home was in Liverpool, was wild with delight when she saw her mother and sister on the dockside. They managed somehow to yell messages to each other above all the din and across the great distance between them. Verna, after much difficulty, made them understand that we were not disembarking that day and her sister, who was very beautiful, called and asked her to ring her up at the office next morning as soon as she disembarked.

"Yes I will," Verna yelled. "What's the number?"

Her sister yelled a number but Verna had to ask her to repeat it which she did, very slowly and distinctly.

"Have you got that?" she yelled.

"Yeeesss," yelled several hundred soldiers. How she blushed and how everyone laughed.

After dinner I took a walk on deck with some of the girls and I think I realized then for the first time that the war was really over. Lights blazed everywhere. England had been blacked out for several years when we left and we had almost forgotten what England with bright lights looked like.

I glowed inwardly. We did not know what was going to happen in the immediate future; there was smallpox on board and the ship was in quarantine, but I was home. The war was over at last and I must learn to adjust to the postwar world. What a glorious adventure it was going to be!

I looked back to that sunny Sunday morning in 1939. It was still very fresh in my mind. So much had happened to me and to the world since that day, but poor old England had taken the worst beating. Could she ever recover from it? Of course she could!

It was like being born again and I felt a thrill of pride because I had been born again into this glorious, unconquerable little island.